Speak Life

Crafting Mercy in a Hard-hearted Time

Gary Gunderson

For information contact:
Stakeholder Health on the web at StakeholderHealth.org, or on twitter at @ stakehealth. The author, Gary Gunderson, may be reached at Wake Forest Baptist Medical Center, 1 Medical Center Boulevard, Winston-Salem NC 27105 or at gary.gunderson@gmail.com.

All profits from the sale of this book go to support the educational work of Stakeholder Health.

Cover Photo: Gary Gunderson, Taizé, France.
Back Cover Photo: Apache Plume, taken by Gary Gunderson May 2017 near the bottom of the Grand Canyon near the Great Unconformity where the Tonto Formation rests on the Vishnu Basement Rock.

First Edition: June 2018

10 9 8 7 6 5 4 3 2 1

Contents

Foreword

Before we speak the language of life, we must choose life. In a world populated with cultures of death, and with so much human effort devoted to developing new instruments for killing, the choice for life needs to be made deliberately. This book by Gary Gunderson is a persuasive invitation to make that choice.

The book represents another major step in the journey of a learning collaborative called Stakeholder Health. A few years ago, leaders from several mission-focused, charitable, and faith-based health care organizations formed a network to share ideas and inspiration for fostering the health of whole communities. It had already become entirely obvious that the approach of meeting our nation's health needs through inordinately expensive episodes of rescue medicine was not sustainable.

Many forward thinking health systems began to look for strategically astute ways to address the complex social factors that are so often the causes of preventable illness and injury. These systems, with a deep heritage in caring for the most vulnerable and marginalized members of our communities, began a remarkable process of rediscovering their founding purpose and recommitting to their historic mission. They were learning again to speak the language of life more robustly. Around the nation, a willing consortium of those who share the vision of equitable and effective care emerged. Several national conferences, two of which were held at the White House, and two books later, this network has grown into a movement, connecting those who want to go far beyond perfunctory reports about required "community benefit."

Gary Gunderson has been the visionary leader of this movement. Beginning decades ago with his widely celebrated book *Deeply Woven Roots*, Gunderson has offered a vision of how life-affirming communities of faith and hope can be transformative. The subtitle of that book, "Improving the Quality of Life in Your Community," testifies to this abiding commitment. The present book gives the movement a mature expression of its sustaining values.

From one perspective, the movement might appear to be merely the sharing of smart approaches to what is now called population health. But a more careful look, with focused attention to the spirit of the work, reveals something deeper and more lasting. It is life-giving joy in the hard work of the journey toward social justice. The real fuel for this movement is the conviction that together we can build communities in which every person counts, where no one is left out, and no one suffers needlessly because of institutionalized unfairness. To speak life, then, is to adopt the ways of life so that every person is celebrated by a community that genuinely cares.

In the broadest sense of the word, this movement is *spiritual*. Though the names by which engaged communities of spirit are known may be innumerable, they share the deliberate commitment to support life. Some of the essence of this spirit is expressed in words supplied by theoretical biologist Stuart Kauffman when he writes, "Our choice is between life and death. If we choose life, we must live with faith and courage, forward, unknowing. To do so is the mandate of life itself in a partially lawless, co-constructing universe, biotic, and human world." The author comes to this conclusion via the avenues of science, not religion. But he knows that the choice for life is profoundly spiritual.

Others, with their own vocabulary of life, come to the same conclusion with the aid of their distinctive heritage of faith. For example, in the tradition I know best, the founding teacher once said, "I came that they may have life, and have it abundantly." Whatever is included in that abundance, it is surely more than simply making a living. It is the composing of a life that matters within community—a life that is life-giving. No single book will be able to present a complete blueprint for such a life. But *Speak Life* will give thoughtful readers plentiful opportunities to explore their own hopes for abundant life, for themselves and for those with whom they share life in community. As the person who chairs the Advisory Council for Stakeholder Health, I am grateful for this opportunity to invite you to enter this conversation and experience anew the spirit of speaking the language of life.

Gerald Winslow
Loma Linda University
May 2018

In the Beginning

"I'll give it all away," said God. That's how it started, with an idea of life. From that first micro-nano of time until the latest Carolina Spring, we have been carried on an explosive, incomprehensive generosity. And when I say "we," I mean a really crazy assortment of life. God could have done it more like one of our faith or hospital committees might: do a controlled pilot project of life on just a small little solar system with less than a dozen planets; with maybe just a few kinds of people who all look and think alike. We'd have kept things polite, tame and predictable. Not the God of this place! Life scattered everywhere, finding its way into cracks we had no idea existed.

The scale and energy of the giving is entirely beyond measure, but since it is happening even on our little planet out on the edge of smallish garden-sized galaxy, it is not beyond our sight.

I wonder why we don't notice it more? I wonder why we don't speak about that? This book does.

And in this hard-hearted time, I wonder why we fall for the scarcity scam nearly every time. Every little despot and predictable tyrant says the same dumb thing: "There's not enough to go around! We must huddle together against.........them! If there isn't an obvious 'them,' they just shout louder hoping we won't notice that the them-of-the-month looks just like part of us. The immigrants! (Who? Except for a relative handful of First People every darn one of us immigrated here.) 'Them poor!'" (Says rich people who haven't broken a sweat in three generations.) Them that don't speak English! (as if Jesus did).

Meanwhile life keeps expanding in a riot of generosity. No matter how tightly the rich hold on, the rest of the planet seems to be inclined to life. You'd think we'd find the courage to give our lives away, too.

I'm like one of the nameless grey neurons way back out of sight whose job it is to connect the signals those many eyes are seeing. I'm not qualified to do very much useful most days, but I am privileged to work among wide, extended webs of those who know what to do in the middle of the night while standing with first responders at a suicide with weeping parents; who build a school for young women in the fire and dust of Kabul; who do surgery, administration, therapy, research and discovery into the mysteries of neighborhoods and molecules where surprising agents of hope can be nurtured. Some of those agents are named Big Dog (the benevolent gang leader in 38109 of Memphis) and R. Ernest Cohn, the Jewish Integrative Medicine Chiropractor who runs a free clinic in Wilkesboro so frugal it borrows its Wifi signal from the tattoo parlor next door. What I see through this collective eye is life, tenacious and fiercely protective of its most tender edges.

Here We Go

This book is about one simple word, *life*. You might wonder whether such an obvious concept can even take up a whole book. Perhaps it seems like I've used a lot of words to discuss something so simple. But even—maybe especially—the most obvious things get lost when we leap to clarity before pausing to respect complexity. This subject—*life*—has gotten covered up with so much other stuff that it's hard to really see it for what it is, even though it is right in front of each of us every day. How is this even surprising? There are so many other things we overlook or forget to remember because they're so deeply buried.

My wife TC and I own a very, very small house in a bit of forest perched on the edge of the Blue Ridge. The sun rises early here, peeking high above Pilot Mountain. Winston-Salem, North Carolina, is 52 miles away. You can probably see half a billion trees. That makes it easy to overlook the one standing 60 feet away. When we bought the property, which used to be an orchard, it had become filled with a tangle of scrub and thorns so thick that not even a deer could navigate it. I was determined to clear space so I could plant some walnut trees, imagining my grandsons Charlie and Asa standing under them when they are old and I am loam. I liked the thought so much that I didn't notice the outline in the corner of the lot beneath the smothering green curtain of vines of what appeared to be... a walnut tree.

The vine is wild grape, which is perfectly adapted to life in the Blue Ridge mists. It's not like kudzu—an invasive species brought from Asia as a quick fix for soil erosion—which can climb up and over anything, turning the noblest of southern forests into big green mounds. Native wild grape is like Southern history, clinging to young trees as they age and grow. As William Faulkner put it, "The past isn't dead. It isn't even past" (Faulkner, 1951, p. 286). It's right there, choking the life out of everything.

I googled "How do you get wild grape off a walnut tree?" Duh—cut the root! I pushed through the brush with my chainsaw to sever a vine as thick as my arm that snaked up and out of sight in the limbs of the old tree. The leaves browned within days after the vine was cut, but the Internet warned me not to try to pull the thick vines out. Google advised me to let a few years pass. The vine would eventually fall out of the tree. But already there was a profound difference: I felt the walnut, now free, taking in the spring sunlight like a newly-released prisoner able to finally focus on life.

More than anything, I want to write simply and clearly about what matters most. It boils down to one simple question: How are we to live in such a hard-hearted time as this? What matters most is that you and me and the other grownups lead lives that are not simply long or wealthy, filled with adventure and pleasure, *but lives that are generative.* We must lend our hands, minds, and time, alongside other humans, to create social structures—organizations, networks, and movements—that are generative. Generative lives doing generative work. That's what we want.

Writing about *speaking* may seem dangerously like walking the long way around the barn, with the whole planet melting right under the feet of our children. Surely we can do something bigger and more dramatic—faster and louder. Tweet something. But what? The most obvious instruction—do not hurl your children to their deaths—doesn't help if we can't tell the difference between the ways of life and the ways of death. We are mute because we have lost the words for life. We have lost our mother tongue.

In the beginning was the Word, says John. We can't do what we can't imagine. We can't imagine without an image. We can't pursue a vision for which we have no words.

When I first uttered the phrase "leading causes of life," which led to the book I wrote with Larry M. Pray titled *Leading Causes of Life: Five Fundamentals to Change the Way You Live Your Life* (2009), I was at a microphone in Milwaukee, Wisconsin, following a profound and utterly devastating message by Dr. David Williams, now of Harvard University, about the relationship between race and death in America. I had approached the microphone with the intention of leading the academic audience in singing "Gonna study death no more." I was thinking of the great liberation song *Down by the Riverside* with its iconic line, "Gonna study war no more."

I didn't do that, but I did leave my PowerPoint presentation and notes scattered on the floor. I spoke—and listened to myself as I spoke—about the necessity of turning from the study of death to the study of "the leading causes of life." I immediately learned something profound: If you only get the question about life right, it's infinitely better than any answer you might discover about death.

A Journey in Seven Explorations

I hope this book is smart enough to be useful in your life and for the world. It's not a detailed roadmap; it's more the way you get directions in the country. I hope you'll recognize the landmarks relevant to your journey. You'll already have noticed a distinct lack of footnotes throughout the text. I've written other books and articles with bushels of them, but I thought I'd keep this text as smooth as possible. I've done the typing for this book, but borrowed and mashed up from dozens of years of working with hundreds of partners. You'll find fairly extensive notes supporting each chapter at the end, including suggestions for further reading that shaped my thought.

The book explores seven concepts over eight chapters; think of them as if in a dance. These are explorations around the idea of focusing on life in new and generative ways that are not problem-focused or fear-based. Each chapter offers examples of how these ideas have been used in practice in the various contexts I've worked within—usually at the intersection of faith and healthcare. The chapters are broken down as follows:

Step 1: Speaking Life

You may speak English or French or Sesotho. You may be bilingual or trilingual—may even speak five or six verbal languages. While we may not always think of it this way, life is also a language. It has logic, grammar, structure, and vocabulary. We need to learn to master it so that we speak it fluently. Like most really important things, this is a lifelong practice that evolves and strengthens over the course of a human life. Keep remembering to speak life. Keep perfecting your proficiency in the language. Practice often; speak life every day, in everything you do.

Step 2: Living Without Boundaries

Speaking life helps us to think and talk in ways that are relevant for our fluid and turbulent times. We left the safe harbor decades ago, but still act as if we can go back to a place that no longer exists. We need deepwater logic now, logic that will help us live out of sight of land, probably for as long as anyone reading this will live. For that handful of readers who have read my other books, you'll see this as a leap beyond *Boundary Leaders*, challenging you to live a generative life without the boundaries we humans tend to like so much.

Step 3: How Life Works

This chapter adapts the logic of the Leading Causes of Life, which has a wide and lively literature. The concepts are radicalized here to serve the demands laid out in the first chapter; we explore how the Leading Causes of Life help us see life working as a complex and generative adaptive human phenomenon. That sounds abstract, but it is actually very squishy. It will help you see your very favorite things—you and those you love—more clearly.

Step 4: Working With Life

This chapter lays out the tools for generative work—the daily normal labor that expresses the logic of life. It opens the toolbox with disciplines of abundance, which includes mapping assets and crafting a "trellis" for things to grow on. The next sections explain how to work with the generative social forms we already have—projects and committees—along with two new forms: limited domain collaborations and *poeisis*. Some of this information will be new, but mostly it invites you to see your work in new ways.

Step 5: Poeisis

In the previous chapter we looked at four basic kinds working with life. One is so distinctive and different in our hard-hearted time that it needs its own chapter. Here work is delight, almost as serious and extraordinary as is play for a child. *Poeisis* is how we work with the very stuff of life and find our selves in the process. But not only our selves—as if they could be apart—but the opposite. This isn't any higher moral plane to get to, and certainly not apart from the grime and grit of doing mercy and justice. But it is the name of how we find ourselves in losing ourselves in the work of life.

Step 6: What Matters Most

Getting the story right encourages and protects the work of life from being sucked back into the vortex of mere problem solving. Life is too important to be left to data collectors and accountants without necessary guidance about what matters most. Accurate accounting, evaluation, and reporting are the key to melting the frozen cultures of traditional power structures so that even they might serve life.

Step 7: Chaos Fights Back

Life turns energy and creative attention in new directions that change priorities. It's not just adding life to something already in existence, like putting icing on a cake. This requires a whole new recipe with different ingredients. The approach is not without risk, especially for those working in organizations built to solve problems—those that take great pride in beating back death. We also have to look out for each other as the chaos inevitably fights back against life.

Step 8: Risk Life

Not to ratchet up the pressure, but the future of the human race de-pends on whether a critical mass of grownups figure out how to give life a chance. We aren't doing very well so far. We have to take bigger risks and pick up the pace. We won't take big enough risks if we aren't crazy in love with a world that breaks our hearts open with its beauty and joy. We need play, delight, curiosity, and *"what-the-hell-ness"*—not ponderous solemnity. Life is the thing that draws us, not just in chaste sterility but in a kind of reckless abandon. Give it all away, but never give up.

Speak life and speak it well.

Gary Gunderson
March 2018

STEP 1

Speaking Life

For many years, our family celebrated Christmas Eve by opening our home to friends whose relatives lived far away and who needed to borrow a family for the night. And then the time came when we were no longer home for the holidays ourselves. Instead of having hundreds over to our home, we threw in our lot with whomever happened to be in a North Georgia Waffle House.

The "A-Team" restaurant staff is not usually covering Christmas Eve, so interesting things have happened. Once we were waited on by—I swear to God—Mary. The teenage waitress was pregnant, unmarried, and obviously ready to birth the Prince of Peace right there in the corner booth at any moment. We ordered eggs, eggs, eggs, and, for me, a waffle. After a bit, the eggs (along with the requisite hash browns) showed up. Waffle?

"Oh, I'll be right back," the waitress promised.

Our coffee cups were refilled twice and each time I mentioned how good a waffle might taste. On the third go-round, the waitress noticed *all by herself* that I was waffle-less. I heard her exclaim (as she shuffled out of sight), "Waffle, waffle, waffle."

You would not expect that a person would need memory tricks to remember *waffles* in this particular place.

And you wouldn't think you'd need to remember what life was about, either.

Robert Farrar Capon wrote *The Astonished Heart,* the title inspired by Ecclesiasticus 43:17-18 (King James Version), which reads: "As birds flying he scattereth the snow, and the falling down thereof is as the lighting of grasshoppers. The eye marvelleth at the beauty of the whiteness thereof, and the heart is astonished at the raining of it" (p. 118). We live in a beautiful world, and we have the capacity to be generative beings, acting out of profound love. Capon continues, writing:

> The Lover who restores the world in Christ is not the God of the philosophers or even the theologians (unless they are very astonishing theologians indeed). And that God is certainly not the god of the inner-harmony-through self-help gurus.... He (or she) runs the world from beginning to end by the radically astonishing device of romancing it into being out of nothing.... And when every last particle of creation— including you, me, the lamppost, and the church—ends up dead, gone, and at absolute zero, its heart will still leap up at the voice of the Beloved (p. 122).

"Waffle, waffle, waffle," my waitress muttered, trying not to forget the word emblazoned on the sign outside. "Life, life, life." I find myself muttering this word all the time. It should be easy to remember—but somehow it just isn't. Not without effort.

Remembering to Remember

It's easy to forget really important things—waffles at a Waffle House? All joking aside, this is especially true when handling thousands of life-and-death events and a couple billion dollars. Take my own institution, Wake Forest Baptist Medical Center. We remembered to put the 35-ton Moravian star on top of our building at Christmas. But… how to say this? We forgot to put up the *cross* during Lent this last year! A former chaplain called, wondering if a policy decision had been made to secularize things: roll the bunnies and eggs, but hide Jesus? Nope, we just forgot. When reminded, up went the cross in about an hour. Even when you have a ground-in tendency to forget, it's easy to remember. All it takes is a nudge.

The Reverend Doctor Susan Thistlethwaite, former president of the Chicago Theological Seminary, said that churches and hospitals should have to qualify before they are allowed to put up a cross. It's not a pom-pom that you wave to cheer on your religious team. It's a signal that you remember that life is found by giving it away; that the most important things cannot be bought at all, but are there for the receiving—grace, forgiveness, a second, third, and fourth chance, all built into the very fabric of the universe by a loving God. And it's a signal that while none of us can qualify as "righteous," Dr. Martin Luther King, Jr. said that we can all be great, because we can all serve. Abundant life is found in giving it all away, especially to the stranger, the widow, the orphan, the poor, the voiceless, and the cast-out. Sounds like an emergency room to me.

A hospital or church doesn't show a commitment to service by putting up a cross. This particularly weird symbol points away from religion entirely. The God of Israel *hated* that religious stuff, as most every god does. The Old Testament prophet Micah stated the obvious: "You know what God requires: do justice, love mercy, and walk humbly" (Micah 6:8). A creed like that will get you killed; just ask Jesus. And it will bring you to life, too. That's what we must try to remember. It involves looking past many of the lies we tell ourselves.

The Illusion of Success

We have had such success at manipulating things, inventing profound and silly stuff, and solving problems—both vast and trivial. Cars (electric to gas and back again to batteries), planes, rockets, fast trains (except in the United States), immunizations, wireless webs, and pills by the trillions. In a very short time, we have gone from not even knowing how the leading cause of death (tuberculosis) spread to largely controlling it, while entirely eliminating other big killers such as smallpox, and soon even polio. It's been an impressive run, but it has made us numb and dumb about what matters most, the thing life itself depends on. Many of us seem to have become mute, distracted by the "things" of success and failing to notice the profound problems that we are not one step closer to fixing.

Obviously, we have achieved much success as a species. Our problem-solving has accelerated to the point where it is now quite possible, if the current trajectory continues, that by 2035 the gross global differences between the rich and the poor will have been largely eliminated. It will take a few more centuries for the nasty disparities *within* each country to disappear, however. It is always easier to solve problems at anonymous range than to do anything about those that are close to home. But it is astonishing to consider that we are only a few decades away from a landmark achievement: average longevity and basic indicators of well-being such as adequate food and water being equal across the species. Not all that long ago,

Jean-Jacques Rousseau considered it a law of nature that three of five children should die before the age of five. Thank God for that broken law. Death rates are dropping and life expectancy is rising everywhere. It turns out that we can do an extraordinary amount of things—even things that have always seemed impossible.

Consider the past 11 or 12 decades during which the average human life has been transformed from a short, capricious, and painful journey of about five decades to a much more comfortable and healthy existence of often more than 80 years, mostly graced with reasonable shelter from the cold, adequate food, immunizations from many diseases, and pills for most kinds of pain.

No wonder we think about solving things all the time. It feels great! Let's do it more! Solving things is like sex, especially the mechanically oriented adolescent encounters that take place before we start to notice the relational nuances. There is a euphoria that comes with solving things. A long-sought-after goal has been achieved! You can hardly think of anything else. You did it! You made it work! It's still working!

Just to be clear: I'm entirely in favor of solving things. I'm in favor of sex, too. But I'm suggesting that we move into later adolescence at least, where we are expected to talk in full sentences about sustained generative relationships that we expect to last for longer than a momentary spurt.

I have spent most of my adult life in some of the institutions most responsible for technical progress, especially progress in the area of health. I was part of the global surge to end hunger. Over the past few decades, the mortality rate caused by starvation dropped from a daily toll of 80,000 children to well below 20,000. (Before you cheer too quickly, imagine a stadium filled with their mothers.) I was part of The Carter Center, a colleague and witness to the grinding progress against polio, river blindness, and other scourges thought invincible. I worked with The Centers for Disease Control and Prevention during the time when HIV/AIDS morphed from a cruel threat spread through the dark and silent shadows of sex, gender, and repression to just another chronic condition manageable with the right pills, waiting only for a vaccine to finish it off for good. I have friends in the World This and Global That. It's all impressive, but fragile—*especially* when the work is mostly technical, beyond the grasp of normal humans.

The Carter Center

The Carter Center, founded in 1982 by former U.S president Jimmy Carter, is a nongovernmental organization guided by a fundamental commitment to human rights and the alleviation of human suffering. Working in partnership with Emory University, the Center is guided by a fundamental commitment to human rights and the alleviation of human suffering. It seeks to prevent and resolve conflicts, enhance freedom and democracy, and improve health. Find out more at https://www.cartercenter.org

The problem is that all this success has not made us *happy*. This is a bit of mystery, but I think it has mostly to do with the vast anxiety engine that keeps revving up our desire for more stuff and to achieve freedom from new and ever-expanding fears. Anxiety is an appropriate response to those who threaten us—who would steal our wallets and votes. But underneath this constructed anxiety lies a deeper disquiet.

Many of the tools and techniques that have powered a vast and rapid improvement in material circumstances for most of humanity have also empowered very old-fashioned instincts to steal from and hurt other people anonymously at great distances. The same century and a half that gave us the end of smallpox also gave us oceans of blood and plastic, along with a radical concentration of wealth and control. There is an unprecedented tidal flow of untethered refugees who can never go home. While we may have the tools to discover life's building blocks floating in intergalactic clouds, we seem to have forgotten the things that make the human life we already have possible here on our perfectly good little blue marble.

Is it possible that the technicians will simply overwhelm the venal elites with a high tide of average well-being? Maybe. So who cares if a few float on yachts for another few decades while we finish getting everyone else clean water? Who needs justice if everyone can read, get on the solar-powered web, and live 70 years or so? We'll finish up the lingering problems of democracy later on. But beating back death is not the same as pursuing life, even when the progress is delivered by technicians with really good manners. We can do better.

The Problem with Problems

The problem with problems is that the most important things are not problems. Life is not a problem. Life is the answer.

Success with problem solving has led many of us to believe that everything can be understood as a problem. We tend to think that a large enough group of experts with enough money can solve anything. We've become so good at solutions that we've forgotten how to talk about the things that generate life.

I have heard otherwise intelligent people actually say out loud that the problem is that we haven't problematized things clearly enough to think them through to solutions. Granted, this is generally

Stakeholder Health

Stakeholder Health, formerly Health System Learning Group, is
a voluntary learning collaborative of some 50 plus participating
health systems and invested institutions calling for operational
transformations that will align with the profound changes occurring
in all aspects in the provision of health care. Its partners share a
commitment to the optimal fulfillment of their charitable mission,
focusing on efforts in communities where health disparities are
concentrated. Participants see in the current policy environment
the opportunity to address the underlying causes of poor health in
their communities by strategically allocating charitable resources,
working with diverse stakeholders to deliver the right balance of
services and investments that improve health, reduce costs, and
contribute to overall economic vitality. The learning collaborative
was sparked by a series of stakeholder meetings convened by
the White House Office and HHS Center for Faith-based and
Neighborhood Partnerships and is administered by a secretariat
housed at Wake Forest Baptist Medical Center. Find out more at
https://stakeholderhealth.org

in a university setting where most everyone is paid in accordance
with the fearsomeness of the problems they claim to be able to
solve. Cancer and heart disease get big money; highly specialized
and obscure diseases not so much. The key, according to this way of
thinking, is to conceptualize one's work as a problem and then draw
a direct line to a group of anxious people with deep pockets. Other
academic disciplines struggle with this since English, theology, and
the classics are hard to problematize. The faculty in these subject
areas hope that the children of wealthy scientists and entrepreneurs

will want to enjoy their subjects as a kind of rebellion against their parents.

Some see life as a huge thicket of problems that will all eventually give way under the glacial advance of the problem-solvers. Should we simply wait for them to sort out global warming and then hope they'll have time to solve our personal challenges too? We don't need their help worrying. Maybe we should spend even more of our waking hours focused intently on all of our personal and interpersonal problems. That is pretty much what we're doing right now anyway. Do we need to do it more?

Life is not a *problem*. Life is the endlessly creative generative phenomenon through which humans find our way. I've only been part of generating two children and now a couple of grandchildren. They aren't problems; they are hope. They are what matter most to me—the measure of whether my handful of years have been worthy or not. One can measure one's entire life by the possibilities fulfilled, not by the problems abated.

Grownups organize themselves into families, neighborhoods, associations, congregations, and all sorts of institutions in order to behave appropriately in the face of the primal possibility—to nurture the next generation. This is the utter and total opposite of problem solving. It is laying down our lives so that the next life has its best chance at moving into the wildly unpredictable possibilities that define humanity.

For the past dozen years I've worked in senior management in multi-billion dollar hospital systems that find a way to give another day of life to thousands of people. I see conditions that until recently meant an inevitable and painful death—diabetes, heart failure, and cancer—now rendered manageable, albeit at vast expense. These huge organizations with thousands of staff manage these illnesses so reliably that most people forget that it is all much harder than landing a robot on a comet. And that has only happened once.

Health professionals can now speak casually of "managing" the health of entire communities, even regions, just as the global summits speak of removing the cruelest burden of poverty from the world. Hospitals like mine have confident committees that work every day assembling computers and protocols and squadrons of health technicians focused on managing the health of the population, most of whom they have never met, and with few of whom they would care to mingle. With such impressive silicon and stainless steel, what could go wrong?

I've been part of broad national and global networks working with dozens of hospitals, world networks of faith, and public health departments. One such network, Stakeholder Health, arose from the bitter ground of Memphis and the toughest parts of other towns such as San Bernardino, California; Detroit, Michigan; Toledo, Ohio; and West Baltimore, Maryland. How do we accelerate the progress of mercy in those places and places like them? We do not lack the techniques, but oh, these humans!

I have worked near some of the iconic leaders of our era—close enough to see them think, do, speak, and lead. These include Jimmy Carter, Dr. Bill Foege, and Don Hopkins, who have saved the lives of hundreds of millions of people and led massive, intricate efforts to eliminate smallpox and polio. I've worked with great hospital system CEOs such as Gary Shorb, who turned Methodist Le Bonheur Healthcare in Memphis from a complacent community hospital into an engine of regional excellence affiliated with the Mayo Clinic.

My favorite leaders work in much more difficult places than any

C-Suite or global summit: those with uncertain budgets, little power, and a bitter history. They just won't quit; they carry on when hope falters. I tune my heart and mind to the witness of people like Larry Pray, a no-big-deal genius who teaches us the ways of life with (literally) his last operational synapses remaining after a string of strokes and heart attacks following a lifetime of diabetes. Reverend Richard Joyner works on the tortured Conetoe, North Carolina soil to find life in those left long behind. June Britt, the heart of Lexington, North Carolina, who is a FaithHealth Connector for Wake Forest, knows all there is to know about racism, but is so tenacious she'll knock on the door of a broken trailer draped with a confederate flag to deliver food to a child of God.

The toughest people know about life, not just death. What if they could work together in generative partnerships rather than fighting the good fight alone?

Methodist Le Bonheur Healthcare
Methodist Le Bonheur Healthcare is an integrated, not-for-profit healthcare system based in Memphis, Tennessee, with locations and partners across the Mid-South. Throughout its history, it has remained affiliated with the United Methodist Church, inspired by faith to serve patients and improve the health of the entire community. Through a partnership with the University of Tennessee Health Science Center, the hospital helps train the next generation of medical professionals and brings cutting-edge research and treatment to patients. It seeks affiliations with community organizations and congregations who work with the underserved, believing that everyone should receive the best possible care. Find out more at http://www.methodisthealth.org

New Kinds of Partnerships

Stakeholder Health has been dreaming up new ways to collaborate ever since the White House came to the tough streets of Memphis, Tennessee, during a blizzard in 2011 and discovered hundreds of dedicated congregations in a covenant with Methodist Le Bonheur Healthcare. An extraordinary learning journey ensued that led through several White House events and other events around the country. What were we trying to learn? We wanted to know if it was possible—and then how—for these institutions to give themselves to the well-being and wholeness of their communities. This learning came to sharp focus last year in a book by many authors, *Insights from New Systems of Health* (2016). It is not imaginary, but a *testimony* to work *already* alive in the toughest neighborhoods. It's all about resilience, obvious but radical new ways of understanding money, and crazy smart ways of doing community health work. It's about leadership, relational technology, global perspectives, and—over and over and over again—about being deeply accountable to our mission. It feels like *life* pulsing.

Those involved in learning know that even vast institutions aren't capable of achieving all that is possible without a fundamentally new depth and breadth of partnership with the faith already alive on the ground. Many hospitals chatter on about population health as if it is something that can be done *to* a passive community, sort of like one might do liver surgery on an anesthetized patient. We seek partnerships not out of etiquette but out of utterly practical need. It's the only way for the possibilities to become realities.

Politicians have always seemed to have a knack for taking religious traditions built for shalom and making them blunt, dumb, and mean. The easiest way to accomplish this is to turn faith against faith—which is even easier if the members of one group have never met members of the other. It's hard to be mean to or frightened of someone in your daycare pool, someone with whom you've eaten and prayed and laughed.

It is now a fundamental competence of the 21ˢᵗ century that anyone in a leadership role in healthcare or public health knows how to engage faith and the structures of faith in partnership in a broad health strategy. But this isn't about memorizing lists of things that different religions are anxious about. It means understanding their generative capacities—how they contribute to the life of the whole.

This kind of movement is not for everyone. Don't come near it if you think faith is best left behind or that the best of faith is behind us. Don't come near it if you think that medical computers and machines can be programmed to create health without needing grownups on the streets. Don't come if you're more interested in death than in *life*. And don't come if you think that your churches and mosques and temples have pretty much done all that your God has deemed possible.

Moravian Brass Bands

Old Salem, North Carolina, where TC and I live, was founded by a group of Moravian religious fanatics in 1752. They were crazy enough to walk from Pennsylvania into a southern wilderness where they hoped to live a life of radical integrity. Moravians can be thought of as Protestant Jews, their similarities including a history of having been hounded almost to extinction in Europe before finding a safe place to live out their emphasis on peaceable industriousness. They are still a bit on the edge of the "normal" spectrum for Christianity, now two and a half centuries later. This is most evident on Easter night at around midnight when brass bands from Moravian congregations all over the city start walking the streets in their neighborhoods, playing hymns as they gradually move toward Salem. They play all night even though not many people can hear the music through their modern sealed windows. Some probably think they are dreaming the old hymns and don't even realize that actual people are playing the music. Hardly anybody knows the words to the hymns. But in the dark the bands can hear each other; as they come closer they tease. One band will play a phrase and then stop, teasing with a tuba. Another band two-thirds of a mile away will pick up the melody. It's not an organized activity, but neither is there anxiety about getting it right; people have gotten it *right* enough for a couple hundred years. Meanwhile in the early dark of the burial ground named God's Acre, a congregation of people gather: people of many persuasions intrigued by the constancy of the Moravians, some wondering about the faith stirring in their own hearts. By dawn, hundreds of brass ensembles have found their way to the burial ground, some straggling in just as the sun breaks over the ridge through the dogwoods and cypress trees that frame the space. It is beautiful. More important than that, it rings *true* in a curiously non-creedal way.

Henny Youngman, the comedian and violinist, once said of love something that is even truer of faith (paraphrased): "You can't buy love, but it can cost you a lot." This movement is free, but it might cost you a lot. It turns out that life thrives when you give it away.

Beyond Leadership

You may be leading a life—your own—and even aspiring to lead other lives, but what you really want is to be led by life. This provides a nearly infinite range of opportunities to express and be part of generative processes. Sometimes you will convene and play roles that look like what others would call "leading." What you are doing is lending yourself as an agent of generativity.

A word you won't see often in this book is "leadership." It triggers thoughts of being in charge of this or that thing, having these or those "followers." I hope you'll focus on leading—but leading your own life. If you are tuned in to how life works, you will be a highly generative agent in your family, neighborhood, and in all the relationships that matter to you.

Life works in the open spaces where pathologies are cleared away, where people find food, where disease is abated, and where girls learn to read. But don't confuse life—the complex creative phenomenon—with the relatively simple process of fixing broken things. Life is an *entirely different set of skills.*

Many of the tools you already have work better in the light of life than in the shadows of death and fear. You'll find that you already have most of the skills you need. You'll also discover what those skills and tools are actually good for. Problems pass when a solution arises; life generates and lives in the possibilities left behind. Problems magnify only what is actual now, in the moment; life magnifies what could possibly come next. Both are equally real: the now and the next. Thank God for problems solved. But how do we think about the other thing, life? The life outside of problem solving?

This question was asked at Jesus' tomb: "Why are you looking among the dead?" *Life* had happened; He had risen. The angel told His followers to go find someone who needed... life.

We have endless ways of defining ourselves, often by our jobs or accomplishments. We need new ways to think of ourselves as agents of life.

Movement Grunt

Most of us can expect to live maybe 30,000 days. We tend to think of the couple hundred days when we are in charge of something as the most important. I was in a big and hopeful meeting at Vanderbilt University, the kind where important things tend to happen. Even the governor was there, along with the rest of us who were not the governor. We had other less impressive roles, but he asked us to raise our hands to indicate our primary profession. The question stumped me, so I raised mine about six times. Healthcare provider? Academic? Minister? Theologian? Activist? Consumer? Not doctor, nurse, chaplain, counselor, or anything actually *useful*, of course. Then a voice from the back of the room called out "movement grunt."

I like it! Although maybe "life grunt" would be closer to what I aspire to be. Being a life grunt involves recognizing that life is not a thing we lead as if we are in charge of it. Life has us, uses us. Being pressed into that service helps us find our own life in the larger life of the world God so loved. And still does.

Amid the infinite complexities of the issues that shape the health of our communities, we could spend time spinning fantasies of solutions that would make things right. We could imagine counsels, committees, and memoranda that would bind together science, ethics, power, and rationality. Maybe we could even... lead these initiatives! All this does is tempt us away from the real work of the imagination. In the end, it tempts us to despair by turning us even more inward toward ourselves.

We are in a Dietrich Bonhoeffer moment (Hale, 2018) that calls for something at once more humble and radical. Faced with the catastrophic collapse of all that was good in Germany, the young theologian formed a small group of people who prayed, read the Bible in big chunks, studied, and prayed some more. Bonhoeffer hoped that the community of spirit called "the church" could be useful for the world. He fell in love and he wrote some letters and a couple of books. (I wish he had written more.) And he gave himself to a violent failed plot to assassinate Hitler, for which he was killed just before the war ended. He did what he could with who he was, what he had, and what he knew. He was not a heroic loner; he was a member of a community of Spirit. He was an extremely well known Spirit grunt.

We know we live in terrible times when we hardly notice the mentally ill under the bridges or sleeping on the steps of our downtown churches. We are no longer sickened by the amputation epidemic caused by uncontrolled diabetes that fills our streets with people on little scooters. We are hardened by the casual violence in jails filled with addicted neighbors. I do not know whether all of your and my best efforts combined will do any better than Bonhoeffer's did 70 years ago.

I do know that we must help each other live lives that are about *life*.

STEP 2

Living Without Boundaries

Crafting Mercy in a Hard-hearted Time

News flash: Life has no boundaries. It's not that it happens out *beyond* the boundaries, but rather that it happens *in between* things that seem to be separate. But no matter how separate they may seem, there is no real separation and no boundaries. If you are fishing, the point is not to organize the gear, but to get into the flow of the stream. You don't want to spend your morning standing on the banks, which merely hold the current. If you are looking for human life, look in between the formal structures, whether they be crafted of steel, credentials, or privilege. This is inconvenient for those who think that leadership depends on getting everything in its place. There's no such thing as getting everything in its place. When there are no boundaries, there's no place where everything needs to be. Leaders who take on this new paradigm have to be prepared to proceed very differently from the way they may have in the past.

The Interfaith Health Program (IHP), where I worked for Dr. Bill

The Interfaith Health Program (IHP)

In the 1980s, William Foege, the Executive Director of The Carter Center in Atlanta, Georgia, and the former Director of the Centers for Disease Control and Prevention, led The Carter Center in work to identify the barriers to the health and well-being of communities and the societal resources that could be mobilized to meet those barriers head-on. Although religious institutions represent one of the most pervasive and powerful of those resources in virtually every community, public health practitioners had not fully engaged the full potential of collaborative networks with faith communities. In an effort to forge such collaboration, Foege enlisted the assistance of President Carter to establish the Interfaith Health Program. It wants to see communities naming their own religious and health assets; public health leaders, practitioners, and researchers seeing those assets, often for the first time; these assets aligned and activated in new ways that enhance the health of those communities; and faith communities and public health practitioners working in partnership for healthier communities. Find out more at http://www.interfaithhealth. emory.edu.

Foege and former President Jimmy Carter, focused on working in the boundary zones between organizations and systems. We found that people who work largely outside and away from the institutional centers of power, lending their lives to improving health in the community—people such as public health field workers or clergy in smaller congregations—often described themselves in negative terms. They saw themselves as being on the margins and hence "marginalized." The IHP, in contrast, saw those margins as places of positive ferment. In these places, leaders are closer to what needs to emerge in response to public challenges to health. The traditional power centers are poorly equipped to navigate the discontinuities so visible in health. They are the problem, not the answer. We see today a broad revulsion with the complicities so often evident at the center. Despair reflects what is missing: a positive life-oriented commitment to life—in the margins.

Moving Through Discontinuity

The great physician Jonas Salk thought that life moved constantly, if not steadily, through states of discontinuity—which is what a species faces when it faces changes that require profound change to ensure survival. In *The Survival of the Wisest*, Salk (1973, pp. 68ff.) observed that the human species had relatively few behaviors that were as hardwired as those of even highly evolved social species in the animal world, such as lions. Their coloring, feet, teeth, and social proclivities and behaviors are perfectly adapted for life in the African grasslands, as any zebra can attest. Humans are not particularly well adapted physically for much of anything: We are slow, awkward, weak, and naked. But we can talk, think abstractly, imagine something new, plan its embodiment, and carry out our plans in creative and often ingenious ways. We are thus capable of social adaptations that allow us to fit into—and even thrive—in many environments. Humans, Salk understood, held this positive adaptive power in their cultures, not in their genes. Culture may not always be quick to change, but it is remarkably adaptable, even if the process of change is often filled with stress. Salk believed that it might even be possible for the human species to exhibit enough wisdom to choose social patterns more fitting to what we now understand to be a closed environment on a limited planet, very different from the open grasslands of Africa where our journey as humans may have well begun.

Salk drew two curves that suggest successive cultural eras, one gently sloping up to a gap (Era A), followed by another sloping away (Era B). He suggested that a species such as ours finds ways to thrive

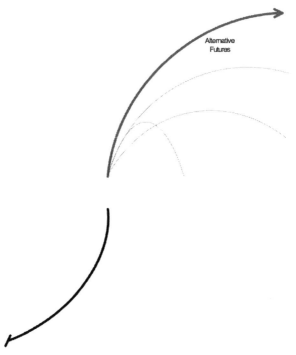

in one era that may be quite different from the behaviors that best fit the next, noting that we currently live in the discontinuity between eras. To a certain degree, we always live between two eras, but some discontinuities offer up a greater challenge than others do. The greater the difference between eras, the more profound the instability, the less clear the path from one to the other. The gap between eras is not just empty time, but a point of inflection in which the path might bend away from the old toward approaches to living that are fit for the new (Salk, pp. 16ff.).

Boundary leadership, a concept I wrote a book about some years ago, titled *Boundary Leaders (2004)*, sees discontinuity as open space in which leadership is possible in ways that are different from the leadership seen in places dominated by systems committed to stability. Instability amid injustice, for instance, is a good thing; it signals a broken-openness within which new things might find life. The point of inflection in Salk's diagram, where one human pattern changes into another, is turbulent, complex, and uncertain. It might be better or it might not. It can be an anxious time, even for those who are more likely to thrive under the new pattern than they did under the old one. The reality is that multiple futures compete for attention. Past and present experiences, events, and actions shape the momentum, trajectory, friction, viscosity, and velocity—all descriptors of change and motion—of future alternatives. Boundary leadership prefers motion over stability. It views the fact that we are not hardwired into fixed behaviors as good news.

More Radical Tools

Alternative futures may be shaped by generative leaders who create new patterns of hope, fear, and confidence. They can also be shaped by a new bunch of well-dressed thieves, so the stakes are high. It is possible to "capture" the whole state apparatus to achieve the goals of a tiny group, as we see happening in many countries today. While these regimes often survive for decades, they always collapse eventually, often on top of the poor.

It is hard to know how large the critical mass of generative agents needs to be for new patterns to develop, but as with other tipping points, that number may be much smaller than one might expect, given the catalytic role boundary leaders play between eras. If (a big if!) their patterns of hope are adapted to reality, they will endure and form new stable relationships. These, in turn, provide the scaffolding for fresh institutions, systems, and culture. Relationships make possible innovations and efficiencies reflecting the multiple intelligences that are needed to find a path toward hope and survival. In the most nitty-gritty kind of way, they help the human community be "fit" for the future or, as Jonas Salk would say, fit for life.

This way of seeing community provided the foundation for a remarkable cooperation between the Centers for Disease Control and Prevention (CDC) and The Interfaith Health Program at the Rollins School of Public Health at Emory University. These organizations, in cooperation, developed a leadership training program designed to shape boundary leaders. For example, 49 individuals in nine teams from Tennessee were trained in three different sessions at the week-long institute. Many of these individuals, if not their teams, continue to play significant roles in the unfolding pattern of faith and health work in Memphis—including me. Ironically for a boundary leader, I found myself in a highly placed role at one of the largest institutions in the region, Methodist Le Bonheur Healthcare. Protected from the delusions of power by the concept of boundary leadership, I participated in the emergence of the Congregational Health Network in Memphis and all its later iterations and adaptations as a reflection and embodiment of the idea of generative leadership.

Boundary leadership, an idea built for discontinuity, isn't quite radical enough to meet the present challenges of leadership in the 21st century. It still tunes the mind toward imagined boundaries (remember, they don't exist!) and leadership (always a distraction). We need stronger language to avoid being tamed to serve the interests of traditional, positional leaders, even those interested in determining the health of such a complex form of life as a "public." We have to test

The Congregational Health Network is a partnership between Methodist Le Bonheur Healthcare and over 600 mostly African-American congregations and other community partners in Memphis, Tennessee. The Congregational Health Network has trained more than 4,000 persons in a variety of community-based sessions designed to build capacity in community and congregational members. Cited as a national exemplar in partnerships between urban, under-served persons and health systems, their work demonstrated ability to decrease costs in early cohorts, compared to matched controls (AHRQ, 2014; Cutts, 2011), as well as decreased mortality and longer times to readmissions (Barnes, Cutts, Dickinson et al., 2014). For more information, see http://www.methodisthealth.org/about-us/faith-and-health/congregational-health-network/.

the words "public" and "health" in the same way we test "leadership" and "boundaries" to ensure we are thinking clearly enough to serve life the best possible way.

Public health, as a field of inquiry, is committed to discovering and explaining patterns and consequences, and has good tools for achieving these goals as long as it is focused on things like germs and risks. But the field struggles with humans, which are infinitely more complex. Perhaps you've met one? We need more radical tools to discern the fluid and non-linear dynamics of social reality. We have found help from complexity theory, sometimes known as chaos theory (the classic introduction remains James Gleick's 1988 book *Chaos: Making a New Science*), which takes seriously the non-linear nature of much of our reality, including the way health works with humans. The language of causes, determinants, vectors, and predictors is so Newtonian—much better for describing bouncing balls than human systems in discontinuity. In a world that can be potentially upset at any moment by volcanoes, fissures a mile under the ocean, and rapidly evolving viruses, we need language better fit for the discontinuity in which we find ourselves. Boundary leadership as a theory and practice only got us part of the way to where we need to be, ultimately stumbling over its two main problems, baked right into the name itself: "boundaries" and "leadership."

Beyond Boundaries (and Leadership)

Boundary leadership was a sort of beta version of what I now think of as "generative agency." Some of you may be more attached to the word "leadership" than to the word "boundary," and it may well take you until the end of this book before you become comfortable with the risk of seeing *your whole life*—all that you do and are trying to do—as the generative agent rather than focusing on the behaviors you manifest when you imagine yourself to be in charge of something. Speak life with your whole *generative* life. But before you just go ahead and pick up a new label, think carefully about the language and what it means by first considering what seemed like really good words: boundary leadership.

Boundary leadership was born in the upland Piedmont region of Atlanta, Georgia, in the academic working environment of a presidential center. The image of the boundary zone was drawn from the vast tidal marshes of Glynn County on the Georgia coast, where every day the tides flow in and out (and up and down by nine or ten feet), feeding a wildly rich ecosystem. This image demonstrated a recognition of the "in-betweenness" of boundaries, their character as places of great emergent vitality: places that are not marginal but seminal, the zones where life emerges.

The problem with boundary leadership was not inadequate conceptualization of skills and behaviors. It has always used a borrowed box of tools. As a former carpenter, I know all about improvised tools. There were times when I swung anything handy (and heavy) in order to knock a grumpy board into place, my perfect hammer lying just out of reach. Many familiar leadership tools work perfectly well, if turned to different purposes than originally thought possible. The skill lies in seeing what to use the tools for. For instance, boundary leadership borrowed heavily from the forward thinking conceptualization of a team of writers who developed a model of "transformational competencies" under the auspices of the Public Health Leadership Institute. This IHP-led and CDC-funded training of teams of both public health and faith leaders to enhance the health of their communities engaged hundreds across the nation in the late '90s through 2009. Boundary leadership took it one more step, beyond the still-parochial identity of "public health" leadership, to declare boundary zones as the home for a new way of leading in general.

Unfortunately, it turns out that the language, if not the idea, of boundary leadership is capable of being tamed. This taming transforms it from a borderland fox into an institutional poodle. Someone in a classic "command, control, and manipulate" leadership role, like an academic dean, might describe him or herself as a boundary leader, though their job is mostly to patrol boundaries and screen anything that threatens the treasures encased within. Just as boundary leadership could borrow tools for more radical purposes, so could boundary leadership be harnessed for more traditional aims. The same tools can be used for opposite purposes depending on the lifeworld—or healthworld—(Germond & Cochrane, 2010) of those doing the talking and those exercising the power. This is where the idea of generative agency might help. This concept is less easy to tame and more fit for the radical turbulence of our current discontinuities.

A River is Not Its Banks

I took a photograph of a river from a plane window near Jacksonville, Florida. From this vantage point the river looks like a kind of line, and it does in fact often serve as a boundary. But you'll also notice that it is anything but stable. You can see where the line used to be and guess where it will move in the future. This is not a bad map to depict a typical generative life—assuming that one can appreciate the nature of the liquid flow we call a "river."

Between Memphis, Tennessee, and West Memphis, Arkansas, a liquid mile away, the Mississippi meanders in much the same way. The concept of generative agency may feel like something from the city of Memphis, which is situated on the mud of the Mississippi River, which drains 42% of the North American continent. This is green but gritty land, fraught with deep historical and material burdens. Many living there are caught in gross disparities that have shaped generations and continue to threaten those to come. Despite decades of investment in health in the region, the overall health profile of the city's population reflects the deep inequalities present there. No matter how hard anyone tries, hardly anything changes. A discontinuity in this pattern would be very welcome indeed. The problems are obvious; the possibilities are not.

John Barry, in *Rising Tide* (1998), describes the Mississippi River like this:

It roils. It follows no set course. Its waters and currents are not uniform. Rather, it moves south in layers and whorls, like an uncoiling rope made up of multitude of discrete fibers, each one following an independent and unpredictable path, each one separately and together snapping like a whip. It never has one current, one velocity. Even when the river is not in flood, one can sometimes see the surface in one spot one or two feet higher than the surface close by, while the water swirls about, as if trying to devour itself. Eddies of gigantic dimensions can develop, sometimes accompanied by great spiraling holes in the water (p. 38).

Liquid reality is far more complex than the land through which it flows. And the complexity of human ecologies, including those linked to health, go far beyond the intricacies of any river. In the Mississippi Delta, four major streams of health disparities are visible even to the naked eye: in the lives of frail elders; among vulnerable mothers and their even more vulnerable babies; among those living with predictable and preventable conditions such as diabetes (usually appearing much too early); and in the traumas of those tangled in severely disabling emotional stresses. (Stay tuned for a companion volume to be published later in 2018 that will unpack these four streams in a deeper fashion.) These profound disparities are carried like debris on a flooding river. The cost to the lives of those caught directly in the currents, and to the existence of institutions in the path of the flood, can barely begin to be measured in currency, in "disability-adjusted life years," or in any other such indicator. Each type of condition that marks the population of Memphis has its specialized analyses, its own guilds, and its own alternate futures, but they all flow in a common social channel that actually offers up a dynamic array of options for trying new approaches that might actually change the health profile of the city.

This is how life works. It duels with chaos, but never gives in to fear. Generative agency embraces the predictable stresses that come with a life spent working in and on the boundaries. However, it does not treat those stresses as problems to be solved. They are qualities of life that invite us deeper into life and the wonder of how it works. Those working to improve the health of the public find plenty of mystery in the turbulent edges of work on the boundaries of health, faith, mercy, and justice.

This kind of life cannot be known from the banks of the river. It can only be experienced through participation in the turbulence of the current. You have to be just a little bit crazy to get into the river. Barry describes the journey of one of the seminal Mississippi River engineers who went down *into*, not across, the river to find the truth of its liquid reality:

> Without light, Eads could not see the river. He felt it. The bottom sucked at him while the current embraced him in darkness and silence. The current also buffeted, whipped, bullied, pulled. A diver had to lean against it, push against it. Unlike the wind, it never let up. He later wrote: "... I found the bed of the river, for at least three feet in depth, a moving mass and so unstable that, in endeavoring to find a footing on it beneath my feet, my feet penetrated through it until I could feel, although standing erect, the sand pushing past my hands driven by a current apparently as swift and rapid as that on the surface" (p. 26).

Obviously, to say there are four disparities is an oversimplification. But this is the way problem-solvers think in order to get a grip on problems—or feel that they've got a grip. It is more accurate to say that *injustice* moves "in layers and whorls, like an uncoiling rope made up of multitude of discrete fibers, each one following an independent and unpredictable path, each one separately and together snapping like a whip" (Barry, p. 38). Although moving in messy tangles, disparities do not evince one current or one velocity. In fact, they have no set course—they are a fluid discontinuity—and, if viewed differently, open up space for the life work of boundary leaders who, wisely, choose to align living assets in ways that nurture emergent patterns of life.

Facing Wicked Health Disparities

In the Mississippi Delta, it is impossible to describe even a short span of decades without accounting for constant reversals of logic and decency. Current reality is not made of the remnants of that which has not yet emerged into order, but is a conflict in real time, between forces both fundamental and trivial. Marshall W. Kreuter, one of the great public health thinkers of the 20th century, once said that some public health challenges were "wicked" in their complexity (2004). He was a bit embarrassed about the moral overtones of this word, but the Reverend Susan B. Thistlethwaite of the Chicago Theological Seminary encouraged him in this usage, noting that the full resonance of the word "wicked" was actually appropriate for describing injustices that have persisted across generations when they did not need to do so.

The four streams of health disparities that are presently coursing at flood levels through the Delta region are each different in important ways. At the same time, they share common social etiologies. Unsurprisingly, many individuals and groups experience more than one disparity— sometimes all four conditions—over their lifespan. Because each of the conditions is currently analyzed and served by professionals whose careers take shape primarily within the boundaries of just one of them, another critical fact is often obscured. The multiple trajectories of individuals and groups who experience the conditions depend on a common web of social assets and on how well those assets are shaped by and aligned with each other.

It is not necessarily obvious to a person working in pediatrics that they have any stake in understanding the social assets encountered by someone working in geriatrics, but they clearly do. It is the work of boundary leaders to move into the turbulent flood of health with a view to aligning these various strands and, given the way health is shaped by social and historical conditions (inequitably), to recognize the congruent need to align common community assets for mercy and justice (usually known in the health fields as "access" and "health status change" respectively). Those practicing generative living are equipped for radical turbulence. They still value a certain level of vital in-be-tween-ness, but are also comfortable with a level of disturbance, fluid-ity, and discontinuity that academic deans might find harder to tame.

Liquid Modern Reality

Generative life is informed by Zygmunt Bauman's (2000) description of modern reality as "liquid"—more in motion than not, and resistant to shape, space, or time. That's only a problem if you think reality has to be tamed in order for us to live. Generative life emphasizes the reality that human phenomena are not just in motion but are in turbulent motion. That metaphor is instructive and important. Turbulence has a rich descriptive language emerging out of the study of liquid and gaseous flows (air moving over an aircraft wing, or liquid through a pipe). People who think about turbulence focus on the edges between moving fluids or gases and the surfaces that constrain them. They don't try to stop the flow, but pay special attention to how and when the flow changes from a smooth (or "laminar") state into a turbulent one (Moin & Kim, 1997). The edge is not in charge of the flow, but it can be shaped to make the flow safe. Generative agents actually *like* fluid social environments and are energized by the possibilities of turbulence.

David Bohm expresses confidence that discontinuity is tolerable because of what he calls an "implicate order" driving large-scale adaptive change. Although any one life, family, city, or people (or galaxy, for that matter) may well end, the greater flow of life moves toward an increasingly complex, thriving, and even beautiful whole. This is what we live for—the confidence that the implicate order will emerge, so we can overlook the fact that in human reality disorder fights back. The very worst humans often seek to capture emergence for their own private purposes. Generativity contests with chaos and in doing so can be tempted to mirror its strategies.

Generative life does not deny that boundary zones are contested and conflicted. It doesn't fear these conflicts either. In agreement with Bohm (2002), generative life appreciates that knowledge at the edge of the ultimate can only be known by going there, not alone but by seeking "participatory knowing." In my earlier work on boundary leadership with Larry Pray, I provided a typology of felt strengths and weaknesses that many boundary leaders working in communities identified with, including, for instance, having very broad networks of very thin relationships. This left them often feeling lonely, despite a thick contact list. Participatory knowing takes away this kind of isolation, replacing it with a community of learners who approach the edge together.

Life Inside and Outside of Organizations

It may be obvious that we need a way of thinking about human turbulence in community. It may be less obvious—but no less true—that we need generative agency just as much inside organizations. The walls of your organization don't actually keep turbulence out or hold it in.

The turbulence of human actions and systems sticks inside of organizational life just as much as it does in tough neighborhoods or difficult families. The intensive efforts mounted to create and maintain orderly organizational systems are just like the massive—and ultimately doomed—efforts to channel the Mississippi River. There are no boundaries, inside or out, which is perhaps why we so eagerly create agreements to act as if there are.

The powerful dynamics within organizational life are the energy of life. They are neither to be feared nor tamed. Generative agents seek to guide organizations toward life, just as boundary leaders have emphasized change in realigning community assets. This is no harder or easier inside than out, which I learn every day on the tenth floor of one of the larger academic medical systems in the United States where I am responsible for creating and maintaining relationships between the formal healthcare system and the surrounding communities for whom its services are intended.

Any generative agent's day job is aligning the assets within their influence with the potential life that is trying to emerge. Assets, whether they appear as solid institutions or liquid networks, are all social and alive. The institutions are also liquid. The networks also have form. In teasing them all into new alignments, boundary leaders offer those in community, as well as those inside their organizational environments, ways to seek health and life simultaneously—or better yet, to treat them as essentially the same thing.

For those working in the context of healthcare, this move toward generativity may clarify many possibilities, even as it takes away the false comfort of the walls formed by guilds, disciplines, and logos. Health organizations—when aligned with community partners—have much more to work with than their simple toolchests of service lines and categorical programs; they can work with life and they can do so systematically, in a deliberate manner, intelligently. But the greatest health challenges require leaders to use blended intelligences that complement disease knowledge with life knowledge. Normal healthcare deals poorly with the majority of health challenges: chronic conditions managed over time outside the walls and reach of medical professionals, multiple recoveries (relational, physical), and transitions (pregnancy, adolescence, job loss, retirement, marriage, divorce, and death).

How can leaders work on the edge of such ultimate wonders? Life leadership begins by understanding that life processes are different from death processes, which follow a relatively simple pattern: Something breaks, wears down, gets run over, or fails, generally from a shortage of fundamental needs (food, water, shelter, basic medical care). In contrast, life adapts, moves, and *chooses* through a rich array of social strategies. Life's adaptive vitality prevents leaders from collapsing into premature simplicity so that they can be accountable for leading toward generative life.

Life is what works. OK. But how does what *works* work?

STEP 3

How Life Works

Against the coldness of all the things running—and winding—down, life is the phenomenon that runs *up*. It expands into every possible crack in the predictable curtain of death. It rises up a generation beyond itself and then another. Life is the thing that goes on. As Jonas Salk once put it, "Life finds a way."

And life is the thing that happens during any of our peculiar and particular spans of years. It is the thing visible in the sprawling gaggles of relations we call "family," each one full of impossibly unpredictable events and personalities. Neighborhoods are alive with still another exponential degree of sustained oddness and light, but also with genuine bonds that grow and tangle and persist even as other bonds weaken and disappear. Life is the word that describes what is going on in a town or city as people—so different sometimes as to be almost unintelligible to one another—do, in fact, find ways to relate to each other. They find ways to pave the roads and decide how fast drivers are allowed to travel on them. They agree on standards for restaurant cleanliness, the rules governing who votes and when, the rules governing who goes to jail and for how long and whether inmates will be fed or treated for medical conditions while there. Life figures all these things out—along with the billions of permutations that emerge out of all the figuring, some having to be redone over and over again as distant neighborhoods and cities make decisions that affect the range of available options. Life is the thing with flags and armies, the thing that prints money, agrees on the language spoken, determines who gets to decide these kinds of things for the millions of people and animals living within the perimeters of what we call "nations." Life does all of that and more.

Life Generates Love

Life generates what we love: daughters and sons—and *their* daughters and sons. This is why we call the groups linked only by genes and the overlapping time they share *generations*. The ache of love is the signal that tells us the ones we love are fragile expressions on their journey back to dust at the same speed given to all of us humans. Even you and me. We knew that. But do we know the thing that creates such loveliness amid the cold stillness?

I am a grandfather, which is to say I am aware of how the thing called "family" sprawls totally beyond the reach of any rational biological, gravitational, or time-centered explanation. Sometimes you see the whole thing all at once through the long lens of tradition and ritual. My grandson Asa was born in San Francisco from the love of my daughter Lauren, who was raised through the love of my former wife and I at Oakhurst Baptist Church in Decatur, Georgia. This church, which was in so many ways my teacher about life and faith, certainly also acted as a powerful life force for both Lauren and my other daughter Kathryn. Lauren was raised with spotty theology, but deep and vibrant relationships. When Oakhurst sent Lauren off for her first play opening off Broadway, a member there, Jake Swynt, recounted how she was always worth listening to (even as a child), as he held her on his lap in the nursery while church went on in the sanctuary above.

A few decades later, after Jake had passed on, I held Lauren's son on my lap, playing a role shaped over four millennia by the Jewish people as the one certain way to mark the time when a boy becomes part of that people. Nathan, Asa's father and an atheist scientist, is the fruit of a Jewish family. His dad, Chuck, was as Jewish as I am Baptist. He passed on the energy of faith, even if, as with Lauren, the intellectual content did not quite make it (so far). No matter the logic, Nathan knew what to do with a son—circumcise him! The *brit milah* is a ritual so powerful that it makes even a room full of impossibly sophisticated and wealthy San Franciscans humble—at least for a few minutes. It makes me humble too. This Baptist was given the most exquisitely humble honor in Jewish life, which is to sit in the "Chair of Elijah," part of the ceremony that has been instrumental to every *brit milah* for thousands of years.

I held Asa as the priest did the circumcision; I raised him in prayers to God that somehow work even when the people listening don't believe in them and prefer their own ideas about how the world works. Rituals are smarter than the people who are part of them; they offer healing as well as novelty. The *brit milah* symbolizes forgiveness as well as honoring a new life begun, washed as clean as a newly circumcised penis. What is being washed, sanctified, and blessed is not the penis but the whole unmappable web of relationships that tie the child—in this case Asa—to thousands of years of people. And now grafting to this tradition like a peach branch to an apple tree, is an odd shoot of liberal Baptists. Who knew that could happen?

Life creates, sustains, and changes the relationships between all the stuff, from all the trees down and across the Blue Ridge Mountains to the soft babies who will one day hold sons of their own on their laps.

Only a few years ago, scientists thought that all human behavior would be explained through DNA mapping. It turned out that most of it didn't seem to be affecting anything, so then they thought it was the RNA. And then we noticed that the emotional context of the mother-fetal dyad was turning things on and off. We now have crude tools just sensitive enough to notice the bond between mother and fetus, as well as the echo of the Big Bang that sent out gravitational waves still rippling billions of years later when we cared to look for them. These tools observe relationships among stuff, and they'll get better. Researchers, for instance, just noticed that those attending a moving theater play will find their heartbeats coming into synchrony and that, depending on the closeness of the relationship, those who experience this will find that they stay synchronized afterward. This is crude, of course, measuring the thumping of the biggest organ. We are on the very dawn of mapping the interweaving of energy and spirit. There is no end to relational nuance among the humans and among planets. But words help us see it, even in our own lives.

A Language for Life

To speak about how life works, we need a language built for three things: 1) relational complexity, 2) creative imagination, and 3) generative intentionality. Human life, in turn, has five causes, five broad forces driving and sustaining it at every social scale.

I have spent time in a tent perched on an exposed granite ridge halfway up from the floor of the Grand Canyon, holding on to one pole with my friend Kevin holding on tight to the other while we both prayed for the continued secure grip of the pegs in the hard shale we were lying on. The wind whipped the rain around and sometimes under the tent, but we knew that as long as the poles held up the fabric that held the space, we would be okay. Think of the five Leading Causes of Life as the poles, creative imagination as the fabric, and the generative intentionality as pegs attaching the whole contraption to what matters. (I'm leaving out lightning for the present time). These are: Connection, Coherence, Agency, Generativity, and Hope.

Connection

There is no such thing as an autonomous human being—one entirely alone, separate, distinct, or apart. We are born because two humans shared their essence through a connection that is not even mostly mechanical. The ejaculatory moment takes up a very small portion of the seeking, finding, and bonding that make up the simple biological part of the human life. Not always, but usually, there is mutuality, affection, regard, hopefulness, and intentionality involved in creating life.

In normal human groups, a child is a signal of the future as well a reminder of every other child. The celebration of a child, marked by the *bris* of Charlie and Asa, and also the baptism of Lauren and Kathryn, creates a bond among the people who regard them as the fruit of a group. The social order precedes, makes possible, and generates the child—the generation. Life is social first. It is nuanced connection.

This is not to say that the connection that causes life fits into the formal nomenclature of approved relationships. These formalities are often designed to contain power relationships that may not be entirely healthy for those living within them. My daughters were raised in a place of worship that honored, elevated, respected, and protected women's voices, often fighting with religious cousins of other denominations in the process. Oakhurst Baptist Church ordained the first white Baptist woman in Georgia, Hazel Grady, not 400, but just 40 years ago. It also ordained a gay man, causing the church to be "dis-fellowshipped" from its Baptist connections, who were afraid even to share their reasons for fear they would be drawn away from their formalities and into the wonderfully messy complexity that apparently God made us to experience.

Connection rests on humility, wisdom, and, yes, love. Stakeholder Health often speaks of the "beloved community" as the guiding image for our work, not just honoring Dr. Martin Luther King, Jr., but sharing with him the sense of wonder for the life that God makes possible even in the most difficult and troubled places. This kind of vision calls out practical human models that assume partial knowledge and murky grounds for collaboration, but begin with hope for what is possible when grownups try to lend their best efforts to nurturing the life of the whole.

The Importance of Language

Accurate language for complex human systems is necessary for meaningful success. Don't try to "impact" my neighborhood; *nurture* it. You'll get a lot further faster. Complex human systems, like complex humans, are not predictable. This is why we live in them as with something beloved, not just efficiently but gently and lovingly. I attended church at Our Savior's Lutheran one Sunday not long ago with Larry Pray. Like lots of other Lutheran churches, it offers up a dozen pages of instructions full of words to read (none of which Larry could absorb in his post-stroke state) and a sophisticated sermon (that neither of us could remember). But we—the social body—baptized a little girl, Gracia Abrahamson, anointing her with Mississippi water and a flood of spirit. The collective body promised—before this baby could understand a syllable—to be with her and her parents through their human journey. This journey, like all of ours, is sure to carry Gracia, her parents, and all of us to places unknown.

Larry, still capable of cognitive feats more important than short-term recall, noted that you don't really need to read a printed program to know what matters in church. You don't even need to remember the names of those who love you, since the most important thing is not their separate labels but the common relationship of which they are part. "We're all one body anyway," Larry says. We can speak the language of life without all the footnotes. "We are born fluent in *life*. It is not just enough. It is plenty." We find our life as we move through connections and meanings and possibilities and hopes. We find it as we generate all that might uplift and nurture Gracia and all she will come to call beloved. We hope for all the things that life means.

Our mental, legal, and ecclesiological categories for naming the ways we are connected are never as nuanced and vital as the extraordinary array of connections in which we find life. As I type, I am listening to two cardinals seek each other through their unique songs, finding a common spruce and then a nearby oak. I suspect eggs are on the way. But the nearby robin—a different variety of bird—is not involved. Human beings, in contrast, have a more eclectic array of possible partners and our manner of being together has served us well over at least the handful of millennia we can track. We thrive in diverse connections.

Human life works precisely because our capacity to connect is adaptive, creative, and resilient. Far beyond the Slot A/Tab B biological sexuality, we have minds built to manage highly nuanced relationships. We can recognize thousands of faces seen only at a glance and remember them years later, associating them with intuitive emotions of trust, safety, or fear. Back when our species roamed the savannah, poorly armed and slow of foot, the males were mostly expendable and interchangeable. Women risked their lives to bear children with huge brains, making the act of generation the leading cause of death among them. Why the risk? How did that work?

In our early years as a species, we thrived in unimaginable vulnerability because that alone could create bonds tough enough for the jungle and then remake them, adapting our connections to whatever possibilities life (and the avoidance of death) made necessary and possible. We don't usually worry much now about being eaten by large mammals. But human life is only more and more expressive of the rich array of connections as gender becomes more fluid, family bonds stretch and snap, both releasing and including— in a word, "blending."

Broken Shards of Unhealthy Connections

Viciously disruptive global technology and economic hits rip like hurricanes through small towns whose lives revolved around textile or furniture factories. Every social role, from father and mother to mayor, is shifted, bent, left behind like the Independent Order of Odd Fellows. Humans form new relationships, adapt old forms to new possibilities, find new ways. Sometimes an entire region is changed in less time than it takes for a child to finish elementary school. West Virginia built several generations around the art and craft of digging coal. At one point, it seemed inevitable that every hill and oak in the state would be leveled. Turns out the trees will long outlast the mines. And the people who built social meaning and structures around coal are perfectly adapted to build new meaning in whole new ways. This is not any easier than facing down packs of wild African animals—an activity that also had a high casualty rate (as in West Virginia, it was probably the men who were most exposed). But difficult as it may be, humans find life through our capacity to connect.

It takes very little light to see the shards and blunt trauma of unhealthy connections, missing or damaging family roles—the long echo of pathological relationships of privilege built of coal in Appalachia or diamonds in South Africa. It is easy to diagnose the ugliness of children's lives in left-behind neighborhoods in the mountains or in cities. Increasingly sensitive longitudinal studies have turned the spotlights on the multi-decade wide-ranging pathological consequences of early childhood trauma. I'm not proposing that a modern American city is any worse than the African jungle 5,000 years ago. But trauma is trauma. How did—how do— children live at all?

It is not just the well-nourished spawn of comfortable nuclear families that make it. Most kids make it, at least well enough to find a life they work very hard maintain and protect. Life finds a way across a vast array of connections. We connect. We live.

Coherence

Humans live because of what we know about life. This has little to do with how many facts we know, although facts help. Not having facts is dangerous, but not as dangerous as the absence of coherence that rests on more than raw power and accumulation. Even a very long list of things that are true is not enough to sustain life if those facts do not cohere in a way that supports life.

Coherence is more than facts; indeed, it is more than a list of facts. It is a pattern that ties what we know and believe and feel and suspect and appreciate and fear into a model of our world that makes sense. That deeply integrated coherence invites us into life. Generative coherence is not merely protective or passive, but active, invitational, and driving. It is closer to active, appreciative curiosity than to the confident kind of "bookish" knowing that makes you sit down to enjoy the view as if it were your own. Active curiosity is highly generative because it constantly probes beneath the obviousness of what exists to find what might else be possible. It never looks at a pile of stuff as a pile, but sees it more as a box of parts that could be assembled to make something new that might do something none of us has thought of before.

Living at the Spirit Level

In their book *The Spirit Level: Why Greater Equality Makes Societies Stronger* (2009), Richard Wilkinson and Kate Pickett explore the mystery of why equality makes societies stronger in almost every way and why inequality makes them weaker. Only in recent years has reliable data allowed comparison across many nations for a wide range of health and social issues, as well as detailed measures of the distribution of wealth both between and within nations.

The big idea is that once a society has reached a certain level of economic well-being (think Portugal or Greece), additional average wealth doesn't make as much difference to the quality of the average life as you might think. Once a person has generally available clean water, safe food, decent housing, and basic medical care, other factors are far more important to happiness and well-being. The most reliable way of predicting the health of a society—or a particular state in our Union—is the degree of inequality between its citizens. It makes sense that poor people have poorer health. But why would relatively rich people in an unequal society *also* have poorer health than their counterparts in a more equal society? People in Greece spend about half as much money as people in the U.S. do on health, but they tend to live about 1.2 years longer. Why?

You'll have to read *The Spirit Level* to fully grasp the authors' answer to the first question. But just look around and you'll probably be able answer the second. In my lifetime, the United States has witnessed huge growth in its economy, but nearly all the benefit has gone to the rich, creating a vast and deepening divide between them and the large number left behind. The United States today is made up of a pattern of citizens with quite different prospects. I write as one of the accidental winners. A public school kid born to a teacher and civil engineer, I went to Wake Forest University back when it was for middle class kids who couldn't afford Duke (or get into the University of North Carolina!). When my parents passed away, they left each of us five kids about $15,000, which is to say we were born to honorable work, not wealth. I've traveled to many countries, and I am grateful for these gifts in my life. I am fortunate. But the United States where I grew up largely exists in the past, as Wilkinson and Pickett point out. This country faces a growing sense of conflict among its citizens, constrained by real limits to our growth and real competition for our privileged status.

While these are big patterns, they are not inevitable or irreversible. For instance, the authors chart the large differences between nations and states in terms of whether people trust each other. In Norway, more than 80% of respondents say they trust pretty much everyone in the country. It is common for coffee shops to leave blankets outside on chairs so that customers can linger over coffee even when it's cold. I've seen people leave babies in strollers outside the windows of coffee shops. They would never consider this odd, dangerous, or foolish. What could possibly happen? Just ask anyone in Mississippi, the state with greatest inequality and lowest trust (17%, Wilkinson & Pickett (2009, pp. 52-3) if you want a list of possibilities. Does inequality itself produce a lack of trust, or does the lack of trust produce inequality? The causal arrow goes both ways, but the result is poly-toxic, producing generational patterns that continue long into the future. Inequality produces distance, which produces ignorance, which produces misunderstanding and more distrust and lack of collaboration, and, and, and, and....

This issue has very practical implications for our work in any community that is obviously lacking a lot of the material stuff we think essential for life. We sometimes focus on "things" when it is actually coherent relationships that make all things possible. Inclusion, invitation, generosity, transparency, flexibility, connectivity—all demonstrated among people dealing constantly with gross evidence of inequality on some of the toughest soil in world. This is what we need to see more often. To give health a chance, build coherence and trust.

Coherence Amid Radical Discontinuity

Not everything is immediately possible, and sometimes it takes several lifetimes of almost unendurable circumstances before some possibilities can even be pursued. The Jewish people, along with Africans and others who have been persecuted, know about this. So do durable minority groups like the Waldensians, who were hunted with the full might of the Italian Catholic powers for centuries. The First Peoples of the New World have a strong narrative of resilience, not a list of tricks for success. Their bitterly tough coherence has permitted them to thrive for millennia even when they were actively baited and stalked, forced onto "long walks," and chased into high mountains and remote deserts. These are peoples held together only by the power of their coherent life narrative. Because life makes sense for them in a way that includes multi-generational suffering, long periods of intense suffering have been endured.

Early in my examination about how life thrives and works, I came across the work of Aaron Antonovsky, a prominent sociologist, through the intellectual generosity of the late Tom Droege. Antonovsky made a profound contribution in his too-short life by framing life, not death, as the real human mystery. His book, *Unraveling the Mystery of Health* (1987), was based on his work in the bitter light of post-World War II Europe. He interviewed Jewish women who had survived the extermination camps and found their way to Israel where they lived through three more wars, losing children and family and neighbors at every stop. When asked about their lives, nearly half said they were OK. *What?* That is stunning to the point of the miraculous—a true mystery. Antonovsky found these women's sense of well-being to be an expression of "coherence," which for him meant much more than ideation, optimism, or belief. He was himself agnostic, which is easy to understand. This kind of resilient coherence lives beneath language in the gut and in between people, in the shared identities that transcend formal flags and ID cards.

Fluid Coherence

As with connection, the more formal and set the identity, the less resilient it will prove during an experience that goes beyond the bounds of expectation. If you think that prayer works and that God always protects His favorites, you will have to find yourself a new coherence when your child is hit by a drunk driver or your deacon shows up addicted to opioids or your priest turns out to have a sexual preference for little kids. Things happen that are impossible to predict or even account for, maybe even to describe. Every great religious tradition has a reservoir of liturgy, scripture, and symbol for precisely these times, offering up coherence on the other side of simplicity. Sometimes we speak of that as transcending, but it is more generative than that; it includes everything. This kind of coherence draws on the full menu of meaning-making tools humans have developed over millennia and adapts them to the most unthinkable modern necessities. Who knows what we'll need once Trump and North Korea and Syria put us through their weirdly toxic blender? Unless all the nukes go off, we'll find our way through to the other side.

Coherence draws on and feeds the full array of mindfulness, science, reflection, and other tools of humility that open the way for clear thought. It is not only received as a fully formed tradition, be it religious or scientific method, but as a gift yet alive with possibilities relevant to what may emerge tomorrow. Coherence causes life precisely because it is adaptive—unconstrained by the past but informed by what has been found worthy by others. These discoveries might turn out to be what we need to be curious about next. Coherence serves life because it *expresses* life; it is still happening, yet it is emergent. It is not finished. Coherence doesn't just happen in the head either. Doing is a kind of thinking; thinking is a kind of doing. The body knows and teaches. The blade cutting the Oregon myrtle spins three thousand times a minute and is a teacher in every sense. You hear the cut and the changing timbre of the thinning shape, feel the dulling edge, smell the wood—so distinctive from oak, cherry, or olive. The body shifts before instructed, a sense of reverence emerges before it is ever expressed. The whole experience of giving form to a simple bowl is one experience—full, rich, coherent.

Generative life is characterized by humility, humor, curiosity, and respect for facts. All of these things can be learned. They all express coherence *under construction*, which is the only kind that lasts, the only kind that drives life.

Agency

People do, act, choose (now, not then; here, not there; this way, not that). They move, resist, play, show up, and sometimes just stand there waiting. Humans are agents in their own lives; they are not passive subjects in the stories of others or objects to be used up. Granted, our species has the longest period of abject dependency of any mammal. We are ridiculously helpless, utterly vulnerable, for a long time after we are born—birth itself being a fraught passage for all concerned. Oceanic biologists have found a species of octopus whose mothers spend nearly two years on the bottom of the bitterly cold sea waiting for the baby to become independent. That seems absurd, except when we reflect on how long we live bonded to our children's every need. It doesn't get much better when they are six or nine or seventeen. It takes a long time to develop the capacity for agency on one's own, but we are utterly dependent on the quality of others' agency in the meantime.

A generation ago, in the dawn of the era of HIV/AIDS, parents (both men and women) were dying at astonishing rates across Southern Africa. The disease flourished in the silent and broken places where the traditional family had been shredded by the migratory labor patterns demanded by industrial mining. Before the disease was understood, the children left behind were feared and stigmatized, expelled from the connective tissue of family and village life. Fear of an inexplicable epidemic overwhelmed any sense of coherence that might have been offered up by science or religion.

Tens of thousands of broken bands of children lived an almost feral existence. In nearly every village UNICEF surveyed, a group of women had, without authority, guidance, training, or resources, simply found ways to provide care to these children. The feral kids somehow found their way to these refuges. Lacking anything but agency, they found a way to live. Now, 20 and 30 years later, the vast majority of those kids have families they are raising in quite different circumstance. Their sense of connection with family and those who helped them informs a coherence born of impossible exclusion based on fears for which science and religion have long apologized. People find a way by finding a way.

Sometimes a group discovers its agency through a powerfully-formed sense of identity and coherence. Such groups are able to fight or love or run or work. But sometimes it is the other way around entirely. Sometimes all is lost and broken apart; however, even in dire circumstances such as these, people will rarely sit down and just watch death approach. We try something and then try something else.

Governments can have agency, too. Franklin Roosevelt waded into a catastrophe beyond measure, logic, or illumination when he was elected president during the Great Depression. This was a depression so deep, broad, and global that no previously useful proposed solution was even in the right weight class. A deep whirlpool of anger, despair, distrust, and sadness sucked like a riptide out beyond the cold breakers. Crippled by polio himself, Roosevelt tried everything he and anyone he could enlist to try could imagine. He invented not only wholly new programs but whole new *types* of programs never before considered. He had too little time to really think any of these solutions through at all. His philosophy? *Just do it. Try it.* Name it anything you like, but just try it. Much of the stuff didn't work, but the trying signaled a kind of tough-minded determination that was otherwise impossible to imagine. The sense of connection that came from trying at large scale created a shared identity—coherence— where before it had been everyone for themselves. The nation became a people in so many ways—a people who found themselves capable not only of survival but of mercy, even a hint of justice. The connective tissue of our people lives long after the individuals themselves are gone—through Social Security, parks, roads, libraries, and deep values that are often only severely tested decades later by those too rich to remember how difficult it once was.

Good Crazy

Joseph Lowery had a beatific love of justice and a wicked sense of humor. He spoke in Memphis at the annual event held every year on April 4 to honor his friend Martin Luther King, Jr. Aging, he told of his son-in-law trying to get him to change his eating habits. Lowery learned about good and bad cholesterol; all fat is not the same. He turned this into a metaphor about agency. "There is good crazy and bad crazy," he explained. Good crazy is when you jump without thinking to rescue someone you don't know from an oncoming subway train (which had happened in New York the week before). One hundred percent *good* crazy. Lowery also described Dr. King as "good crazy." Dr. King would have loved this, an echo of a speech he gave December 18, 1963, at Western Michigan University about creative maladjustment. He said that "there are some things in our social system that I'm proud to be maladjusted to, and I call upon you to be maladjusted too. I never intend to adjust myself to the viciousness of lynch mobs; I never intend to become adjusted to the evils of segregation and discrimination; I never intend to become adjusted to the tragic inequalities of the economic system which will take necessity from the masses to give luxury to the classes; I never intend to become adjusted to the insanities of militarism, the self-defeating method of physical violence." Good crazy.

This contrasts with *bad* crazy, the unreflective, instinctive, and impulsive acts of violence against others, often at the risk of one's own life. You don't have to find a terrorist with a bomb-laced vest to see an example of this. You can find it at the other end of the pew in your church where ancient and stupid ideas are left to fester, waiting for an unhinged moment of meanness. Crazy as a grenade without the pin. *Bad.*

Humans are agents of our own future, built of life or twisting toward death. We don't have ultimate agency to bend reality to serve our interests. But we do have agency enough to find our way. When the Jewish people were lost, broken, without a clue about the future, Micah left his vineyards to point out the obvious: "You know what to do: love mercy, do justice, walk humbly." Love actively; do, walk, and you will live. Still works.

The Power of Generativity

Life finds its way because it out-generates the predictable maladies, frictions, entropic drags, and blunt blows that appear along the way. Life is carried on the current of generativity. Sometimes the current moves like a flood, other times it lies deep beneath a frozen phenomenon like a glacier that seems stationary, yet moves.

The most notable quality of young children is how they play with life. They grab, twist, taste, pull, poke, sniff, and wrestle. They *play*— and in the process they learn how gravity works and how muscles work, too. They figure out how to move this flapping thing with fingers within grasping range of that bunch of Cheerios or maybe the tail of the cat. They play with words until they find sounds that get the attention of nearby servants (such as a grandfather). A blindingly fast couple of decades later they may be playing with ideas, some sort of ball, chemicals, or lines of code in much the same way. They give the unknown a crack in the universe to squeeze through. Generativity is like play but the stakes are higher: life or death.

The essence of generativity is found in the billion choices grownups make to protect and nurture, to make it possible for the young to stay alive. These choices could be characterized as irrational sacrifices made against the logic of survival by the largest and most powerful of the species. There are reptiles who eat their young, and we sometimes hear of similar patterns among the children of divas. But most of the other 6 billion of us give our lives to our young at every opportunity as long as we breathe. Dr. Joyce Essien, an Atlanta-based pathologist, reports on a community survey of a group of poor and vulnerable elders. "What do you need most?" they were asked. The answer, difficult for a group of geriatricians to process, was prenatal care and sex education. "Don't worry about us," the elders said. "We're worrying about these young girls with nobody to protect them." That is normal generative behavior for grownup humans.

What often escapes need-oriented surveyors is the simple truth that what humans need most is to give ourselves to something other than ourselves. We find our lives through giving our vital essence to others. This doesn't diminish us; it fulfills us, propels us, generates our own lives in the process of nurturing others. This isn't even noble; it is the way life works. It's what we're for, how we live, and how life lives.

Generativity is all about being in the right relationship with those who have given to us, to those whom we may be in a position to nurture, and to those around us who could benefit from our choices. We are most alive when we are aware of being in those kinds of right relationships, especially when they find resonance with each other. I have written before of the last years of my mother's life, which she knew was closing on her. She had promised to stay until my book was finished and then added some months to see the *great* grandson who turned out to be Alex. She asked me—told me—that I would do her eulogy, not because the preacher was unknown, but because he was. She wanted to know not just *what* I would say, but which grandchildren would read which scriptures in what versions. I promised to write it all out so in case I broke down and was unable to continue the preacher would have no room to ad lib. We sort of rehearsed it all sitting on her bed with the old Phillips Bible I had marked up in high school. I was crying and she was laughing. The day came for her—as it will for me. At the funeral, I made it pretty far into the eulogy and then handed the slip of paper to the preacher, joined my family, and wept again—not in rehearsal this time. Kathryn, who was 7 going on 70, put her hand on my knee and whispered, "Daddy, you've been a good son today." I am still blessed by that moment, generative across time.

As I was writing this book, TC, my older brother John, and I drove across West Virginia to the other side of Cincinnati where mom had passed her last years under the care of my older sister, Judy. Now it was Judy in a memory care unit, sharp enough to know the pain of what was missing from her mind. John, a catalogue of bad decisions and worse luck, was not much better off, though he was 5 years younger. Judy had not seen either John or me for some time and had never met TC, so we had no idea what to expect. We drove through torrential rain across the high mountains, which took our minds away from the uncertainty. We arrived a bit before lunch and found Judy well enough for a trip to Wendy's. Afterward, Judy made eye contact with me, grasped my hand, and said, "I'm afraid. Don't leave me." She needed me and I needed to be needed. We basically held hands for four hours until she fell into a deep sleep in her bed.

And then we drove back to North Carolina, where John passed away only two weeks later. He was determined to "finish strong" and live into the relationships that mattered the most to him, which is exactly what he did. He was a man who lived by grace and needed a very great deal of it, thanks to a difficult web of anxiety, depression, and alcohol. He never complained or blamed anyone. He wrote poems every single day of his life, and was always working on another novel. He found his life and his ability to endure by being generative.

Life Flows Through

Generativity makes room for the life to flow through. The flow is life-giving for all involved. It is easy to be distracted by stuff. Money, hamburgers, college tuition, cars, food, cell phones, and shoes. This is the stuff and clutter of the 21st century. We need a lot of stuff, or so it seems. But there is stuff we really *do* need, and it is always in the form of relationships made up of various degrees of trust, kindness, and respect. The qualities of the relationships are what provide the life.

A relationship is generative to the extent that it is intended for life, not taken up out of a sense of obligation or domination. This is easy to see in a family, especially among relationships in transition where separation is often marked with energy and friction. The kids are seeking escape velocity, but need fuel. The parents are seeking liberation, but need assurance as their power gives way to love. There is a shifting current as the flow finds a new channel.

Something like this happens in any human relationship. The greater the asymmetry of power, the more the relationship crackles with energy around the qualities of respect. All staff in Wake Forest Baptist Medical Center's FaithHealth Division are being drawn into the weird and often brutal world of the county jail these days, as we provide spiritual and emotional care for the Sheriff's department, where two thirds of the employees work in the jail. As we care for them we are drawn closer to those they protect. We have learned that most of the violence that happens in jail has to do with perceived disrespect, especially between jailers and inmates. Whether it is a pill or a meal or a phone call, if it is not given in respect, it is likely to cause damage. Even when the right things happen, they are generative only if they build the relationship. The same thing happens with public assistance or free healthcare or "special" education.

The challenge is that the arts of respectfulness and right relationships are often lost in the minds of the powerful as they focus on stuff instead of humanity. Inexperienced jailers don't know enough about the lives of the incarcerated, many of whom struggle with substances, mental traumas, and the constant rain of bruises of race, language, and poverty. They don't know enough to have empathy, much less how to employ the arts of human commonality.

Generativity finds the vital way between, among, through, and with. Never to, at, over, or apart. Generativity creates the space and means for life to flow where it will. Life always wants to flow.

Hope

We can go without food for days and water for a few hours. We can't make it to lunchtime without hope. It may be that the whole human experiment is about hope.

During a grim moment in American democracy a couple of decades ago, I ran into Glenn Henson, the most profound ethicist of his generation. Hungry for his hopeful wisdom, I leapt to the most intimate question I could imagine, like a starved man might a leap at a burger. "Glenn, do you believe that God would actually permit humans to end the whole experiment of life through nuclear war?" Back then we thought we were all there was in the universe, so the question was really about all life everywhere. Glenn observed that the question of whether we would choose life or death is really what the whole experiment is all about. God may be curious about whether we can even tell them apart. There is no way to think it through; some of us are born on the light side and think we'll pull it off. Others are on the dark side and tend to think we're doomed. The data seems to favor the ones in the shadows, but life still, against all odds, tends to find a way.

An Inconvenient Hope

It is a curious characteristic of our time that we exaggerate the hopefulness of silly technical advances while refusing to take seriously the evidence of profoundly positive shifts outside the realm of technology.

Dr. Christoph Benn knows the face of suffering up close. He was a physician practicing in Tanzania at the beginning of what came to be known as the AIDS pandemic. Driven by the quiet power of faith, he did not blink at the devastating reality he faced. One thing led to another, and he is now serving as Director of External Relations and Partnerships at The Global Fund to Fight AIDS, Tuberculosis and Malaria. He is now not blinking at another stark reality: By the most profoundly obvious measures, of peace and health, the world is...*improving...a lot* (Benn, 2014). What is the faithful response to *that* reality? Silence, mostly. Since 1990, death rates from disease and violence have dropped nearly in half. *Repeat: Death rates from disease and violence have dropped nearly in half since 1990.*

A striking blend of technology and social/political mobilization involving public, private, and hybrid organizations has mobilized tens of billions of dollars in quite novel ways. These efforts almost always involve religious networks and organizations. But to a stunning degree, religious leaders have hardly known what to say. For the most part they—we—say the same thing we said 50 years ago when we faced a post-colonial world with highly concentrated medical assets and vast impossible demands for basic primary care. Or what we said 100 years earlier, when germs were first beginning to be noticed and we could finally do more than lament. Or perhaps even what we said 1,000 years earlier still, when the world was almost entirely unpredictable except for the certainty that most lives were short, brutish, and painful. This is, Dr. Benn suggests, intellectually and theologically irresponsible. We have faithfully taken Jesus' throw-away comment, "You always have the poor with you" (Matthew 26:11, English Standard Version), to suggest that He was describing a universal constant like gravity, instead of a cheerful footnote on why it was—and is—OK to celebrate the gifts of friendship and fellowship with occasional extravagance. Do you think Jesus or *any* religious leader would give license to mere *symbolism* toward the poor? Not in a world capable of changing in quite fundamental ways. We need not be satisfied with symbols. We can be accountable—deeply—for bending the arc of justice as much as it will bend in our span of years. And it can bend a lot more and a lot more quickly than we may have thought. We can do this thing called justice to the point where the injustices become the outliers rather than the norm.

This is almost as inconvenient a truth as the melting icecaps. What makes global warming an inconvenient—not tragic—truth, is that we can see clearly that we *could* choose life if we *would*. Benn is very aware of the environmental headlight at the end of the tunnel. At the moment when humans have discovered our capacity for *generalized* justice, we could also discover that we have turned our wonderfully made home into an overheated and "unliveable Eaarth" (as Bill McKibben, 2011, now spells it). But if we can make the social choices that have led to such radical declines in disease and violence, we can surely make the environmental choices that would make our common life possible. We are far more likely to make the complex and lengthy choices necessary to forestall climate change if we think the world allows for such basic successful choices.

Perhaps the easier (if previously inconceivable) social and policy choices that have had such success in the fields of peace and health could encourage us to believe in the possibility of making and sustaining the right choices about carbon and climate. I say this as a Prius driver who recycles everything and brings my own bags to Trader Joe's—all the while knowing that my carbon footprint is probably far greater than that of my parents. My environmental symbolism is a kind of complicit despair enabled by the fact that I don't really believe it *can* be different. The successes of global health and peace challenge that complicity. It *can* change, so I *must* change.

The International Religious Health Assets Program rests on a similar warm-blooded view of reality that systematically notices the wild abundance of tangible and intangible assets exactly where you don't expect them—in the tough towns on the northern rim of Zambia, in the delta mud of Memphis, and in the left-behind factory villages of North Carolina. Look and you will see how much we have to work with. Many of these contexts are animated by faith, though it is frequently a faith more obvious to the laypeople on the ground than to the leaders in the pulpits. That simple observation has driven an appetite for a more vital description of faith, spirituality, and spirit that is more like energy and less like a brittle list of constructs.

The voice of faith is too often trapped in a script more suited to the time before germ theory, primary care, immunization, and systematic research into the social influences on health. Dr. Benn, speaking to a mostly United Methodist audience in 2014, noted that the most profound moral energy behind the global health breakthrough on *universal* treatment for AIDS, tuberculosis, and malaria has reflected the prophetic voice of gay men more than traditional faith leadership. Religious leaders (and I'm one of these) were satisfied with doing the best we thought possible, not what science and public policy actually made possible. Can the voice of faith give us courage and wisdom to change a lot more than we thought we could? *Of course it can.* But our view of the world needs a fundamental reset. Otherwise we end up lending our silent weight to the shrill, mean, and small voices that chant, "There is not enough and will never be enough for justice to be a serious choice." Their faux realism assumes a world that forces us to choose those who look like us over those who do not. The world we *actually* have is more like the one Dr. King called beloved.

Beyond Optimism

The hope that drives life is not optimism. It is certainly not false happiness based on a flawed understanding of the fragile limits and boundaries of nature, the nonnegotiable pull of gravity, of fire, and of the need for water and food. We are tuned closely to this very particular physical world, not to Mars or Venus.

Hope is the active ingredient in every placebo ever tested and every behavioral modification scheme for employee wellness that seems to work until it is recognized as a behavioral modification scheme. If you are told that your doctor is smart and that the pill he has prescribed you will work, it probably will, even if it contains nothing but sawdust. Hope is so powerful to our species that even a shadow of it—mere optimism—creates a biochemical response just like "real" biochemistry. Hope is just as real as anything else, because humans are bio-psycho-social-spiritual creatures built to head toward life. Hope for humans is as essential as feathers for birds, so maybe I'll give Dickinson a break ("Hope is the thing with feathers" is a poem by Emily Dickinson, 1862).

The hope that draws humans toward life—that causes us to thrive—is not optimism and it is certainly not about our individual longevity, wealth, or success. Grownup hope is about those to whom we are connected, those with whom our deepest sense of how the world holds together resonates. It illuminates our capacity to do and to choose, and includes our desire to give it all away so that life flows through us into those who fulfill our deepest hopes.

Two Additional Concepts

These five concepts driving life are an ensemble, not a list. They are inseparable, interactive, relational. They each create space and lend energy to the others in ways that make the whole dynamic, adaptive, and smart. Life is capable of becoming *more* alive and then more alive again. These five words will take you a long way toward seeing life where you'd least expect it and will show you how to nurture it where most people would be ready to do an autopsy. But there are two aspects of life that I didn't understand when I was first starting to figure all this out back in Memphis. Let's turn quickly to them so you can see the whole ensemble come, well, *alive*.

Creative Imagination

Humans can think of things that have never existed before. We can just make things up entirely. And then we can act as if they were possible, making the long series of creative choices to give those possibilities a chance to work. Or not. Most things don't work, but that doesn't bother many of our species. We'll just think of something else.

Jim Cochrane coined the term *prosilience* to fill this hole in our vocabulary. *Resilience* looks backward, hoping to restore a condition experienced before injury or to strengthen the capacity to resist damage amid stressful conditions. *Prosilience* looks forward and builds forward to strengthen the potentialities on the other side of stress or injury. Life out-generates pathology; it doesn't just repair. It builds forward. The body and the mind learn from the stresses and injuries of one's life, discovering the kinds of things they need to survive in the future. My own body has learned from when I tore my hamstring clear off my hip that it needed to grow back *stronger* than before, because I am highly likely to do it again.

Much of what passes for creativity is just mashing things up into new combinations. Humans put things together that create new things able accomplish ends that neither of the original items were ever intended for at all. The Black Panthers mashed together a semi-militarized racial resistance group with a soup kitchen and invented a whole different model of radical pride-based social animation. I almost typed "social service," but it was mashed-up with the Black Power intelligence of the Panthers. It is not "service" in the old do-good model, but something entirely other, something generative, different, and alive. The Panthers imagined it by doing it, and turned themselves to acting on their hopes as soon as their creative imagination could see the possibilities.

The Panthers didn't know anything about what I call the Leading Causes of Life and were mostly just angry as hell at the recent centuries of continuing slaveholding-type oppression, some enabled by the taming effect of social services. I doubt they would have even appreciated the positive language of the Leading Causes of Life. But they were *all about* their connections and the desire to break free of disabling entanglements. They were focused on rejecting every kind of received narrative that did not lead to freedom and life. They never missed a chance to seize and express their agency, power, and active deliberate freedom to choose their own way. They were willing to lay down their lives so that others could live. They crackled with hope and confidence, believing that history was bending their way, vital and unstoppable. They didn't swagger out of desperation, but out of hope that what mattered most, even beyond any of their particular lives, was strong and durable. Their claim of life made them free; their freedom made room for creative imagination that powered all the causes of life. This is how it goes when it gets rolling.

Creative imagination puts the causes in motion and lights up the possibilities for where it might express itself next. It sees connections in methods that offer new possibilities that have never been conceived. What if every church adopted one prisoner and loved her endlessly? Jesus died a criminal with two other convicts; why not bring those saving connections back where they belong? Yikes! Connections can be dangerous when reimagined.

Creative imagination sets old ideas, identities, privileges, and patterns afire, burning away the dross and keeping the gold. What if hospitals were organized—found their coherence—around the things that produce health? But, but, but, how will we pay for the beds we already built? "It's only castles burning," sang Neil Young (1970). "Let the dead bury the dead," said Jesus. What would we do if we were all for life? Let's imagine that and see if leads to more life along with less death. That's the whole point.

Creative imagination takes the knowledge of death and links it to our knowledge of the things that lead to life. But it does not treat them equally; it is radically biased on the side of life, giving less comfort with less patience to grownups who refuse to share their vitality with the family members and neighbors who need it. I get mailings from the American Association of Retired People (AARP) more frequently these days and notice that not a single paragraph has ever been about the needs of anybody but old people. The purpose of an old person like me is to diligently give myself away so that the next generation has the best possible chance of thriving. That is my purpose, the whole point of my life. Creative imagination is about visions of the whole, the durable vitality of what comes next, not me and my list of needs that are actually hardly ever needs at all. Creative imagination thinks of life and more life, not just my little life.

Creative imagination holds up hope and makes it a vivid possible choice. It takes hope from an abstract desire, the most predictable aspiration of a grownup looking at the eyes of those who will live beyond them. And it turns hope into a moral claim, an actionable possibility, something that might happen if we acted like grownups who are part of life. Hope leads to life when we have the imagination to see how our little lives might be involved. Fully alive grownups make different kinds of collective decisions when they imagine the lives of those they love having a real claim on their privileges. Life choices face the city council, or—almost impossible to creatively imagine— the U.S. Senate.

Sometimes a quiet constant pattern of doing the right thing, constantly curious about how much right could be done, opens possibilities that nobody really thought possible. This freedom creates imagination. Imagination points the way to express freedom. All my adult life I've been within range of people working on large and nearly hopeless problems. I worked for years on "world hunger," so I still wince every time some finance guy chirps during budget season, "Let's make some real decisions; we can't end world hunger." Turns out we can. We can immunize pretty much everyone. Provide clean water, too. And educate all the girls. Most people can't imagine these things, but the fact is that they are already well underway. We'd have to decide to stop. Who can imagine doing *that*?

My daughter Kathryn gave me a tie that depicts a sliver of Vincent Van Gogh's painting, "The Starry Night" (1889). The outrageous pulsating energy of Van Gogh's stars was part of what got him classified as deranged back during his lifetime; well, that *plus* cutting off his ear and gifting it to a lady friend. But the fact is that those who think that stars are teeny weeny little bitty dots of pale light are the ones detached from reality. They are all—including our own little sun—impossibly vast, distant, and wild pools of energy throwing light and energy beyond our capacity to measure them all across the universe.

The universe may look stable, contained, predictable, and cold—but only until you have the tools to see the reality of a jumping universe. Anyone who has really paid attention to a neighborhood, much less a city, much less a region or a country, knows that is true, too. Who is crazy here?

Generative Intentionality

Generative agency needs one more thing to distinguish the ways of life from death. We have to choose wisely, and, as Jonas Salk (1973) noted, that capacity for wisdom is not hardwired into us. This lack of hardwired wisdom is crucial to our capacity to adapt to radically different circumstances. But it bets the boat on our ability to be wise enough to choose life for the whole of humanity and not for our little tribe alone. We just have to be intentional.

The generative capacities that permit us to hope for life also work just perfectly when bent in the service of perversely self-serving movements. Humans are not hardwired to be wise, but—much better actually—we are *totally* hardwired to seek life with a reckless and eclectic curiosity. We are not wired for much of anything at all, except for the creative freedom to give ourselves to horrible, cruel phenomena as well as to the most noble of virtues. The dynamics that created the institutions and momentum toward a fundamental change in the life prospects for billions of people happened in the exact same decades that saw the rise of the Nazis in Germany, apartheid in South Africa, and the Killing Fields of Cambodia. We are currently dealing with North Korea—and any number of other destructive forces. Intensely connected, internally coherent movements with highly focused agency aimed at generating sustained energy in service of an inwardly focused hope...*work*. Even when they aren't working for good.

I wish I could say that these kinds of movements fall apart quickly, easily giving way to the generative powers of mercy, justice, and life. It turns out that they can last a very long time and do terrific damage while they do. Given the fragile nature of our shredded global systems, shouldn't there be something stronger than the Leading Causes of Life? I don't think there is. Life is all we have to work with; it's the *only* thing that works.

The difference between life and death turns on one question: whose life are we seeking? Mine, yours and mine, or the whole of life—everyone's? Seeking our own life against the whole is futile because of the radically interconnected nature of human and natural systems. You can co-opt the logic of life by focusing on tribal ties against the whole of humanity. You can build a sense of coherence by emphasizing group particularities against the broader commonalities. You can build agency with violence, wealth, and force. You can turn generativity inward, at least for a time. You can prop up a hope apart from the world. It will not lead to life, for that is not how life works. Every empire, clan, corporation, or religion that has attempted these methods is dust, their triumphal bleats written on tablets in a language only the wonkiest historian can even read.

Meanwhile, life finds a way, always testing itself in humility, asking the central question: Am I living for the life of the whole, or just for me and mine? It is the common wisdom of the saints that we find our life by giving it away. This works for larger social realities, too. A nation that seeks its own dominion will surely lose its minor privileges. A religion that seeks its own victory over others will lose its credibility. A discipline that promotes itself against the coherence of all learners becomes a squawking distraction left behind and speaking only to itself.

Seek life and you will find it. Give it away—all of it—and you will participate in life forever.

It works. Now how do we work with it?

STEP 4

Working With Life

L ife is a gift. And life is a craft. Its craft rests on the disciplines of abundance with which we craft generative social forms. Do we have time to learn those crafts with a planet on fire? We cannot know the answer to that question with any certainty. We do know that we have no time to do the wrong work. And we have no time to do our work poorly.

Generative Crafts

Gerald Winslow, director of the Center for Christian Bioethics at Loma Linda University's School of Religion, is the son of a German immigrant house builder and has been a master craftsman of wood for decades. Jerry recently took me over to the Gamble House, in Pasadena, California, the epitome of American Arts and Crafts style architecture built in 1908. It is a revelation in simplicity. Every single joint, lamp, door, handle, light, stair tread, and attic beam was carefully considered and then crafted to express a perfect blend of form and function. The two architect brothers, Charles and Henry Greene, were part of a vibrant global movement that saw in craftsmanship the hope for democracy, the possibility of human culture to make a difference. This was no small thing to believe amid the turn of the raw and violent century when industrial bigots had their way nearly unfettered. Something as modest as a well-crafted cottage might seem hopelessly irrelevant against an unstoppable tide of crass exploitation. But not if that cottage—or chair or perfectly-made lamp—is an expression of integrity, consistent with a whole system of relationships to other people and the created order. What if such people were to outnumber the mean and crass ones? Sounds like question for our time.

In fact, the craftsman movement signaled what mattered most: how to live a worthy life and live it well. Iconic architect Frank Lloyd Wright said of the movement: "Do not think that simplistic means something like the side of a barn, but something with a graceful sense of beauty in its utility from which discord and all that is meaningless has been eliminated. Do not imagine that repose means taking it easy for the safe forest, but rather because it is perfectly adjusted in relationship to the whole, in absolute poise, leaving nothing but a quiet satisfaction with its sense of completeness." (Wright, 1908).

It is time to craft our common life with the same thoughtful attention to form and function as our earlier teachers lent to working with wood and stone. Some of the old tools work fine, if freshly sharpened. Jerry still uses tools he acquired decades ago, sharpened so many times they are a fraction of their original length. Old social tools still work, too. In the aftermath of the recent electoral meltdowns, the Democrat Precinct 601 of Forsyth County, North Carolina, met in the Single Brothers House & Garden in Old Salem, North Carolina, where democracy has been argued for a couple of centuries. We elected a new party precinct chair, who looks for the entire world like Bernie Sanders' granddaughter, but who also knows the craft of elections. The first job is to get acquainted, have a party for the party, read some books, and talk like humans who are capable of caring and thinking about what matters.

Modern tools are important, too. We need to craft messages through relational technologies like Twitter that are too powerful to leave to the mean and desperate. The craftsman movement has a challenge in figuring out what to do with industrial machines, but democracy is played for much higher stakes than any lathe. Respect the medium: watch the density and grain if on a lathe; watch the pattern of need if crafting public policy. If you don't love the wood or the people, go do something else less important.

When there was much to fear in a culture lost to mere machinery, the craftsman movement trusted thoughtfulness and beauty that comes from integrity and a well-lived life. These democratic and communitarian values stayed alive in the culture, expressing themselves later in the practical compassion of the Civilian Conservation Corps (which turned Jerry's German immigrant father into a craftsman), as well as Social Security and policies favoring religious hospitals and non-profit health insurance. They crafted institutions that removed the abject fear of penury from aging and made it possible to fight a skirmish, if not an outright war, on poverty itself.

All the things that hold us together can fall apart. The habits of democracy are not hardwired into anyone. But we have seen worse bluster fail before well-crafted policies and institutions built by people no smarter than us who simply wanted their lives to be good. They even left some tools behind that just need to be sharpened, to be put to the grain by hands who know what their lives are for.

Disciplines of Abundance

A discipline is a set of practices designed to produce a way of life. Some communities of practice are held together over many decades, even centuries, by their discipline—by what some orders call their "rule." You will not be surprised to find that I am no great fan of discipline in the sense of boundaries, prohibitions, and containments. I *am* committed to a body of liberating disciplines that underlie and enable generative agency. Here a just a few suggestions:

Go to the Boundary Zone

If you want to find life, go to where the future is breaking open, where things are breaking and broken. Then pay attention. Go to where others don't want to go; it won't be crowded.

The most important thing to remember is that you're not starting anything. Life is already happening everywhere, and will find a way to continue even if you don't show up and help out. Every job will find a hand. Every sermon will find a voice. In one sense, all the world needs from you is your six billionth. Don't be the kudzu in the garden of flowers already growing by blundering in and taking all the light. At the same time, be aware that most things that happen reflect a small set of active ingredients, rather like the contents of an aerosol can. Your six billionth may be the active ingredient. So put it all in; don't hold back.

The boundary zone in any ecology is the dynamic place between zones of relative stability. This is the tidal marsh, neither solid land nor open water. This is the edge of the forest, neither meadow nor quiet dark beneath the old growth oaks. This is the neighborhood where things are broken open, broken down, maybe breaking through. Generative process is about the new, which needs some open space, at least a few cracks in the pavement for novel possibilities to have a chance. So get out of the castle and head to ground with people who aren't afraid of breaking.

The kind of power you find in a castle can push things and stop things, but it can't *generate* things. It has already paved over the possibilities and is entirely dependent on grazing on the possibilities that may emerge on the other side of the moat. I happen to have an office on the tenth floor of a medical castle filled with decent people organizing things and repairing thousands of lives every day. This often demands exotic and highly honed skills entirely focused on doing the right thing for the person right there. This is the stuff of nobility, done without breaking a sweat. But the people who excel at such exotic work can't be expected to also invent a truly new way of doing entirely different things outside their walls. That happens out in less settled neighborhoods where the ache and grind of change is underway.

It isn't hard to find places where *possibilities* are not exactly obvious but real all the same. These are places marked by vulnerability and the vitality of those who won't quit or walk away. Here you find the edges sharp. You could get shot (probably not), but there is certainly no risk of boredom. All the data shows these places in bright red, as all the negatives converge into a wicked thicket; the charity care, and the lack of high school graduation, and the violence, and the poor housing (and, and, and, and, and). Each of the problems magnifies the next, which is why a generative agent begins with a radically different question. *What is already alive here?* How are those living assets connected? How are they already resonating in some pattern of meaning? How might they find new alignment that would release their resonating agency?

Look for Dynamic Patterns

If you are part of a hospital or helping institution—say a jail—follow your most vulnerable patients or clients back home to their neighborhood. You're looking for *patterns*, not just that one particular person in one particular home. The clinician needs to make eye contact with that *one* human; you need to make eye contact with the context. Map your charity care and then get in a car and drive around the census tracts where that care is concentrated. Get out of your car and walk around, maybe even talk to some people. You are probably not going to be comfortable doing that by yourself, so ask the magic question: "Who am I related to who is related to these neighborhoods?" You know the answer to that question. Often that person will have a uniform; they may drive an ambulance. They will provide further connections. They'll know the name of the pastor who has never been on TV and who doesn't have a sanctuary you'd notice from the street. You will want to get to know him, too.

When Methodist Le Bonheur Healthcare's Center of Excellence in Faith & Health did this in Memphis, we mapped the homes of people who had received charity care, which clustered in neighborhoods where we had already developed covenants with churches. The covenant preceded the data, but it turned out that the churches that shared a curious heart for the poor were concentrated in the neighborhoods where the poor were concentrated. So the data illuminated the value of the webs of trust we already had. When we asked one of the founding members of the covenant, Reverend James Kendrick, if he knew of any neighbors who were patients of the hospital a few miles away, he laughed and organized a group of deacons to go with us for protection. We met Emma, who was living in an apartment complex in one of the few units that had not been burned out by competing gangs, and she offered incomparable wisdom. Emma had had a stroke a few years prior and had difficulty walking, but was intermittently cared for by her niece and nephews, a member of one of the two competing gangs. She still loved her neighborhood, despite homemade bombs setting what little was left of her apartment on fire regularly and the violence swirling; she wanted to stay in the only home she'd ever known, in Riverview, Kansas.

When the CEO of Methodist Le Bonheur Healthcare, Gary Shorb, saw the maps with all the houses in the neighborhoods surrounding the hospital, he wanted to see the streets himself, so he went with a couple of our chaplains to meet Reverend Kendrick; later he brought his whole leadership team to spend a morning at Kendrick's church. A whole program, "Wellness Without Walls," grew up in those neighborhoods, protected by the same gang members who had been asked to give advice. Years later, the roots transplanted into that rugged soil are still growing, even though Emma is no longer alive and Gary Shorb is no longer the CEO of the hospital.

Large institutions, such as hospitals, schools, or jails, are seen, at best, as therapeutic nodes. They are places designed to heal or change something. I know I'm being a bit generous in thinking of jails as therapeutic. But they are by far the largest provider of mental health services in our society. It takes a little creative imagination to shift from seeing them merely in terms of what they currently provide to what they might generate in the future.

You don't need a hospital; any jail will do fine as the way to cross boundaries. Wake Forest Baptist Medical Center's FaithHealth Division provides spiritual care to the sheriff's department and other first responders in Winston Salem, North Carolina, which brings us into the heart of the boundary zones. The heart of the darkest shadow is the jail, which sleeps just about the same number of people every night as the hospital, about 750 citizens. They spend an average of three weeks of the worst days of their lives there. Or maybe not the worst. Half are already living in the shackles of addiction, bruised enough that somebody has diagnosed them with mental health issues, often serious enough to require pills. They are, with a few exceptions, poor. They are overwhelmingly from minority backgrounds and trapped in some kind of substance dependency. Until recently, the jailers were themselves sort of in jail, assigned there as a punishment. Most of the prisoners have been inside before, often with more experience of incarceration than their young jailers.

Dismemberment and fragmentation happen in any place where discernible difference translates into advantage. The distinguishing characteristic may be skin color, language or dialect, curl of the hair, or religious practice—sometimes a combination of characteristics. Sometimes a phenomenon crosses over socially constructed boundaries, which is what opioids did when the prescription medications available to whites resulted in an epidemic among people not officially thought to be vulnerable to addictions. The social body is not confined within communities of color, so the medical professionals doing the prescribing needed to see a new and larger social body—and act appropriately. They (we) can't heal dependencies from a distance. We need to see human commonalities to even begin to understand the mechanics of an epidemic such as the opioid crisis.

Even before we came to see the commonalities between the new and the larger social body, the dynamic nature of the drug trade took advantage of yet another social blindness. Most of the overdoses are not resulting from prescription abuse, but from new wrinkles in the old-fashioned drug market. We are actually a global social body connected in real time by the Internet and FedEx, allowing Fentanyl to flow like poison blood. The chemistry of this particular social disease mimics the rush humans are tuned to need that normally comes from intimacy, love, and connection. A chemical episode ("overdose") signals a more fundamental drive that can't be reversed—humans need each other and will find a way to die when disconnected. The social body needing connection is the whole body, the intimate dyad, family, neighborhood, community, and those creating the relational structures that connect at the scale of the global internet.

The dynamic nature of life gives us eyes for what is still possible for the social body. This triggers the second shift in posture and attitude—from dispassionate objectivity to affection, even to love. Now you need to rev up your creative imagination in order to see the flow of people through the jail, noticing where they come from and where they will go next, the whole cycle of incarceration.

Look Out the Back Door

A generative agent will look not just *at* the door but *through* it. He or she will look at the 25th day of the average 24-day jail sentence. Who is involved in the next phase of the lives of the people you are serving? Every organization has a defined space for its services. Normally, you define the quality of your work by how well you do inside that space. A jail has extreme boundaries, but they are crossed quite quickly and completely when the sentence is fulfilled. A "good jail" is not defined by what happens inside it, but by how well it is integrated with the other institutions and social assets that pick up where it leaves off. Quality is defined by integration into the network of providers, not just by autonomous siloed services. In order to measure your internal quality, you have to look out the back door and see what happens next.

You'll see that those days are part of a long narrative with chapters set in the most predictably broken parts of the boundary zone. If you ask, you'll hear about earlier chapters, often involving enough childhood trauma to break any grownup's heart. Don't look away. Ask the preposterous question: What is possible in these lives? Does life have any chance at all? Feel the six billionth of the human heart beating? Look around to see if there is anyone else also standing firm, not looking away. They'll be there, probably waiting for you.

Go to the broken places and find the live generative nodes of possibility that are already there.

When I came to Winston-Salem, I found a city full of churches and highly visible preachers. Maybe too many. In our little county, the IRS estimates that there are 770 churches, but which ones care about anybody other than themselves? I have generally found that about 10% of all the visible places of worship do 100% of the heavy lifting. Maybe 20% are active in anything that could be broadly understood as relevant to health. About 5% are mean; you wouldn't want to go near them. About half are drifting like plankton with the tide of the post-Christian, post-industrial, post-Constitutional culture. Given the cultural climate breakdown underway, most of these can be thought of as dead churches singing.

There is great news buried in what may seem like a depressing bit of arithmetic. First, you don't need to do anything about the plankton; let it drift. And all you need to do with the mean churches is to stay out of punching range. Focus on the 10%, the heavy lifters, and maybe some in the next ring of those compassionate enough to aspire to lifting something heavy, too—perhaps another 10%. Maybe they have never done much of anything, but under new leadership they are finally ready to become their best selves. In our county, that means looking for 140 congregations with heart. What does it look like for you?

Ask the Poor

Ask the poor whom they trust and find those individuals. Let them teach you. I asked the four former housekeepers who had agreed to lead the way as our Supporters of Health whom *they* trusted in their own lives. In 2012, I was called to be the "spiritual cover" in a meeting led by young MBAs in shiny Italian shoes designed to save the Medical Center a million dollars by outsourcing our environmental service workers. I immediately said, "No—you guys are going to get me fired." My job is to build trust with the under-served and about 60% of our housekeeping staff lived in our top poorest zip codes. So, I made up a deal on the spot to train some of our environmental service workers to be community health workers. The original Fab four (as we called them) led us onto the streets and into the lives of those they knew in ways impossible for me or most anyone in the privileged halls of the hospital to know. I asked the Supporters for the names of the 20 pastors they trusted to care for the poor. I was not entirely surprised that I had never heard of 16 of them. I was even less surprised to find missing some of the pastors most famous (among white people) for their leadership roles in town. Religion is a funny business, but less funny if you're poor. It took several months to meet everyone; many were working as pastors only part time. The rest were pulled every which way into the lives of their most vulnerable members and neighbors, doing more funerals than they had members. I had nothing to ask or promise, so the appointments were often rescheduled. As I learned, I began to see the neighborhoods through the eyes of those who had never looked away.

When you start to notice the reality of life in tough places, you will be tempted to leap to your default scheme of fixing things before you've even really thought about what's possible. You will be tempted to use old ideas and words for new work. This tethers you to the past rather than allowing you to live as an agent of generative possibilities. Be careful how you talk, especially at the earliest stages of entering new places. You don't want to waste new energy and intelligence by doing one more lap around the same old well-worn path. Ask your city planner how many community improvement plans have been done in the last 50 years. They won't actually know the number because it's a big one. The only difference between the earliest and most recent plan will be the name of the dominant pathology—it will absolutely be something bad. You need to do something different, so learn to use different language.

Look for What You Hope to Find

If you are standing in a neighborhood looking for assets, you'll find problems. If you look for problems, you'll never find the assets. Each living thing has two wolves, one of fear and one of hope. The strongest is the one you feed. You feed hope by looking for the assets.

The fearful wolf is the one used to getting all the food: the problem industries leap into action, writing grants in a blink. The heroic problem-solving part of our brain will kick in, too. Sometimes the fear wolf dresses in sheep's clothing, wearing all the trappings of generosity.

Premature, uninformed generosity will crowd out work that

strengthens the life of the community. It will settle for making people feel better instead of actually helping their vital strength. This is stealing the light and energy that could have helped their life grow, strengthening the agency of the helpers instead of the agency of those helped. You will be like the wild grape vines that stole the light from my walnut tree. Wild grape vines—and helping organizations—don't climb up into the light on their own bodies. The native wild grape *rides* up as the tree grows, then spreads out along the branches competing with the walnut leaves for the sun. The walnut isn't exactly killed, but it is stunted. And the whole forest looks silly, more like a grape tree than a noble walnut. *Don't be like that.* And don't let the community look like a forest of helping organizations instead of a living neighborhood of vital social structures.

In the very first Interfaith Health Program (IHP) publication, (*Faith & Health*, 1993), President Carter wrote an article containing the line, "We must make the choices that lead to life." It was an accurate image, rather than a deductive fact. But we didn't build the program around the question by first asking, "What do we mean by life?" That question came much later, after I moved to Memphis where the question was part of the conflagration of hundreds of covenant churches. The question of life was very different in a city far too familiar with death and pathology. It was a positive shock for a hospital executive to approach networks of pastors who knew about death and were used to being constantly asked to enlist in yet another program about some pathological phenomenon. Life? What?

Like me, you're aware that you are standing on sacred ground with a beating heart. That tingle you feel is called life. Just as you look for the pattern in the data, you also want a map for the ground so you can clearly see the terrain, what's alive on which streets. You want to understand the webs of relationships that link the assets, out of which come the possibilities you want to nurture with your own life. This is the explosive disruptive power of mapping living assets.

Mapping Assets

Disciplines of abundance rest on a thoughtful and appreciative inventory of our assets—both tangible and intangible. Then we need a clear-eyed examination of what we could do with them.

The most generative abundance is found in the relationships God's spirit constantly moves in and through us to create. God is connected to everything and everybody. The connections among God's people—all those who turn toward life—are not just abundant but infinite. This is surely the abundance that we have been most undisciplined in utilizing.

You need discipline when mapping strengths and assets because you find yourself drowning in possibilities. Where fear asks us to subtract and do less, hope provides us with more than we actually know what to do with. In the 1870s, Memphis suffered a series of Yellow Fever epidemics that killed at least 8,000 people—more than 20,000 in the Mississippi Valley as a whole (Crosby, 2006). The city of Memphis almost died as a result of bad water—while living on top of the greatest freshwater aquifer on the planet. It is possible to have access to an abundance of resources and still fail to use them generatively.

Over the past quarter century, a number of methods have evolved to make visible and actionable the assets of communities previously thought of in terms of their needs and deficits. This is, unfortunately still a minority view. Legally, the government almost always requires hospitals, banks, radio stations, and such to do *needs* assessments, which trigger the predictable missionary reflexes and whimsical charity that selects from the assortment of needs on display as if choosing a "queen for a day."

South African theologian Steve de Gruchy always said that you can't build a village out of what it doesn't have. Any serious strategy rests on a clear-eyed view of assets. Steve led the development of the techniques used by the African Religious Health Assets Mapping Partnership (ARHAP), which is the taproot of the model described here. ARHAP wove the foundational techniques laid out in the book *Appreciative Inquiry* (Cooperrider, 1999), the organization Asset-Based Community Development (developed by John Kretzmann and John McKnight), along with the rapid assessment tools of African rural development, insights from African sociology of religion, and a hefty serving of hard-won post-apartheid intelligence about the role of trust in large social scale movements. What is now called Community Health Assets Mapping Partnership (CHAMP), a working group built on the U.S. field sites for ARHAP, is a rich stew with a Memphis accent and some Carolina sauce. It was integrated into the population scale mobilization strategies in both settings. It is both an art and a craft drawing from a deep intellectual well.

This model is complex. It was learned through practice, not by reading books. You may wish to use a simpler, handier tool to turn on your imagination locally. Anything that involves looking for assets is better than anything looking for needs and deficits. Read the following to provoke a simple question: *What do we have to work with?* This is a technique designed to blow open space for creative imagination about generative possibilities. It requires four moves:

- First, figure out who cares enough to be relevant to the fears that have drawn your attention and to the hopes you have for what might be possible. Many people will already be taking action, providing some kind of service.

- Second, convene this group in a structured dialogue to create a new map.
- Third, listen carefully and systematically to those *seeking* services or help. Never trust a map that has not been validated by those living on it.
- Fourth, bring both groups together along with others you discover along the way to see if the new map is accurate enough to allow for new kind of journeys.

There is a high art as well as a lot of low, mundane work involving yellow Post-its, Sharpie markers, and large rolls of paper. People need lots of systems and crafts in order for the gift of new insight to emerge. But people are built for this kind of emergence, so something meaningful almost always comes of it.

This is tactile discovery that a computer simply can't accomplish. There are a number of Internet-oriented companies that will offer to "scrape the web" and generate an impressive list of social service agencies for you. They will not actually know anything about them that could not be discerned by looking out of the windshield of a car while driving through a neighborhood, probably less. A person in a car can at least notice the neighborhood setting and whether anyone is waiting outside.

Hidden Relationships

A map of assets is about human relationships, not stuff. This triggers what Tom Munnecke of the P2P Foundation called "the problem of toasters and cats." If you put 40 toasters in a room and come back an hour later, you can predict what will happen. If put 40 cats (or people) in a room for a day talking about the possibilities in a rough and ragged neighborhood, thère is no way to predict what will happen. So the CHAMP process is built around a series of carefully crafted exercises designed to systematically bring into view the long timeline, including shocks and traumas, and web of flow among providers and their current array of locations and networks. Those who seek health on the same map go through a process focused on gaining insight into the weighted trust and value of what is available through the actual journey of gaining access. Same map, but very different views. A third meeting is needed to respond to the blended map.

In Winston-Salem, after seeking a general map of health-relevant assets focused on the five zip codes marked by high levels of charity care, we did four mapping exercises in English and then tried a few in Spanish. Whoa! A good process is one that results in a surprising map. This was a *great* process, opening our eyes to the reality of the undocumented with such clarity that we could not close them again without just walking away. We did not walk away.

We came to see that our undocumented patients faced profound health vulnerabilities because the lack of validated identity documents made it unsafe for them to access healthcare except in the case of a severe emergency or a non-negotiable event such as the birth of a child. The lack of identity documents means that the father's name is not included on the birth certificate. Twenty-first century medicine is not anonymous. It is highly tuned to a continuum of care, typically with a pharmaceutical aspect that allows for management of the condition over time. We had to figure out how to align the range of community assets that might be relevant to *that*.

Trust Validated Maps

The mapping process creates images of possibilities built on real assets that are accountable to each other because they jointly created the map. Those on the map are accountable to focus on it, not to look away from their own map. The imagination moves toward action organically, but not inevitably. Seeing the lives of the undocumented clearly in the middle of the Trump phenomenon is highly inconvenient, especially to public officials and government-sensitive institutions such as hospitals.

A dialogue crafted around what *exists* creates data, evidence, and validated information that has weight. Findings emerge from a process of unquestionable integrity, including discussions with the range of providers and seekers who add additional dimensions of credibility. The sophisticated documentation of the process should be available after being vetted for accuracy by all the participants. The truth tells itself, without anxiety or pretense, and with all participants serving as both actors and audience. There is transparency.

Much of what passes for new thinking about health was laid out by John Wesley in his book, *Primitive Physick Or an Easy and Natural Method of Curing Most Diseases* (1761), written hundreds of years before germs were "invented." The reason it seems fresh today is not because we have new machines, but because we have the possibility of new *relationships* of high capacity, capable of thriving at scale. Keep repeating these words: *building capacities for scale*. This requires what is now possible: rich interconnection between systems for food, mobility, the more complex systems of legal and illegal substances, and the almost infinite array of systems relevant to emotional and mental balance. Oh, my! The challenge is the opposite of what you'd think: too many partners, not too few.

Life Needs a Trellis

There is hardly any example of human life that is not social; the extreme rarity of hermits proving the point. A solitary human is highly likely to be unhealthy—a danger to him or herself and probably others. To work with life, we must examine how we grow together, how we help each other find light. Think of the trellis.

A trellis is built to fit the plant it serves. Its purpose is to help that plant find the light. Plants just need old sticks. Tom Peterson, communications director for Stakeholder Health, tells me that there are at least five million non-profit organizations in the world today, most of them created in the last half century, and almost every single one formed to do something somebody somewhere thinks is useful for improving their community. It's *way* more interesting than that. Many more millions of for-profit companies have been formed in this same time period, each hoping to make money, but also to do something good in the process. Just check out kickstarter.com to get an idea of the superabundance of ideas that exist right now.

The ecology of human forms of association is rich, complex, interconnected, and constantly adapting at the speed of electrons. This is terrific if you need lots and lots of relationships. It is daunting if you think someone should be in charge of organizing them. Former Surgeon General Vivek Murthy (2015) did not aspire to organize 5 million of anything. But he did and still does hope that they (we) can organize ourselves in ways that can make it more likely that 21st-century science (including, but far beyond everything Wesley knew about) can get into the lives of people and neighborhoods.

A trellis is not a miracle; it's just a useful object that supports the miracle of photosynthesis. It makes it possible for plants to do what they want to do—bear fruit. The gardener (and the movement organizer) trusts the process, but doesn't make the process do all the work. I like wine, and I know that good wine needs just the right soil (developed over many thousands of years) and just the right rain (which depends on picking just the right valley and sun, not too hot and not too cold), so that magic happens. But it helps if the vines don't just run every which way on the ground. Grape growers have developed a near-perfect science of trellis design to fit different varieties of grapes.

Emergent social life is more complicated than grapes—and right now we have vines running every which way. It would help if we did the humble work of building some trellises on which could grow a rich array of relationships to bear the fruit the Surgeon General imagines possible. There are four main kinds of trellises:

Conceptual. Stakeholder Health emerged as a learning group that collectively created a monograph to map the conceptual trellis on which healthcare systems could fulfill their missions. It is really good, but like other kinds of conceptual trellises, it needs to be rebuilt for a new season of work (stay tuned at *stakeholderhealth.org*). The learning community will need to be much larger and even more interdisciplinary than the intellectual gaggle that created the first trellis. It will need to build a relational trellis on which to grow (and prune) those fruitful concepts.

Programmatic. The Surgeon General's call for broad activity is not a call to do 10,000 different things, but to find alignment around four things that could be transformational. Thousands of us can find a coherent understanding of our work as linked. Nobody is exactly in charge of it, but a well-built programmatic trellis helps us to find power and meaning in contributing to a very large collective change.

Institutional. The YMCA is made up of 3,000 local organizations whose role has changed quite radically from that of shelters for young men to iconic suburban fitness conglomerates. Now the organization is changing again, embracing its extraordinary role, which is aligned with the Surgeon General's vision. There are many other examples of old structures finding new relevance. But in every case, it is tough work. The 3,000 YMCAs have 900 local boards!

Narrative. Humans live by story far more than we live by objective data. A movement with capacity and scale needs a narrative trellis so that each of us, in our many roles as members, leaders, citizens, and healers, can locate our personal story in the thread of a great narrative. We need the bards, writers, and artists to help us tune ourselves to resonate with a greater tone.

The trellis is logical, structured, well designed, and sturdy precisely because life is none of those things. Life sprawls all over, never missing a chance to try growing someplace else. That's why a trellis is necessary if you want wine from grapes—and why humans need social forms to channel the energies into sustained communities.

Life Moves With Elegant Simplicity

Before we begin looking at forms, I want to suggest that life moves with elegant simplicity to achieve sustained vitality. The work of life, when done well, is hardly work at all. Dr. Paul Laurienti, a brain researcher at Wake Forest School of Medicine, is the Leading Causes of Life Fellow who taught Larry and I to approach life lightly and with wonder. He raises orchids to keep his sense of wonder fresh and often brings an especially beautiful specimen to a meeting and sets it in the middle of the table to let it speak for itself. Paul turned his research on the brain upside down when he turned away from the laborious pursuit of the mechanics in between the synapses to look at how the whole thing worked as a complex system—maybe the most complex system of all.

Paul also uses birds as a teaching example, showing a short video of the murmuration of Scottish starlings. It is a mesmerizing image of complex beauty. The starlings dance in the sky forming patterns beyond words. Thousands of birds swirl, dive, and rise in three dimensions, rushing, but with utter ease. Wondrous. They are all starlings and they know how to act with each other. Humans are less elegant—hard to watch most of the time. We are not alike; Rev. Dr. Kirsten Peachey, of the Center for Faith and Community Health Transformation, says that human neighborhoods are more like a dozen starlings living next to a hawk that eats starlings, next door to a horse, a pig, and a potato. Not quite as pretty as hundreds of birds flying in a pattern. Or maybe it just takes longer for us to identify our common energy. Ben Wolford (2014), writing about the starlings for the *International Science Times,* claims that the way the birds dance is managed "by constantly avoiding collision. Generally, they were taking their lead from the bird directly in front of and below them, rather than the birds to the sides or above."

If you can't understand how that metaphor applies to humans, you have never been on a committee. Heather Wood Ion, founder and president of The Epidemic of Health, sent us another video about starlings, this one showing what happens to a murmuration when a hawk screams into it from above, scattering the birds every which way like confetti in a hurricane. In their bird-like persistence, they go back to regular life; not letting the hawk turn them into something else. They find their pattern, regain their social structure, which is a kind of aerial trellis, and go on.

An Astonishing Abundance

In the past handful of years, astronomers have found that the ingredients for life are astonishingly abundant in places beyond counting at distances beyond imagination. The vast reaches of reality are swirling with the ingredients of life. The places once imagined as impossibly cold and hostile are just waiting for the right relationships to emerge. Life is still finding a way—even in the barrenness of post-constitutional Washington, D.C. It turns out there is a richer array of the basic ingredients than we'd been led to expect. Life at large scale is a tapestry beyond the design capabilities of any of us. The pattern is woven of nothing but incomplete threads, some broken, others full of knots like a fishnet repaired after heavy use. To see it in motion demands more than reason. It demands curiosity and great peripheral vision.

Tom Peterson has been my curious learning partner for nearly 40 years, remaining one of the most lively and eclectic minds in my life. He never ceases to discover new ways to learn. One year he decided to turn walking his dog Wiley into a new form of discovery through the simple discipline of strolling through a different neighborhood in Little Rock, Arkansas, every day. Wiley sniffed around and Tom took it all in. He paints and finds new form and color where nobody else would even notice them. He let his backyard go un-mowed for a few years, just to see what would emerge over time. He observed the lawn every day, noticing each new plant that found itself at home. He stuck to the daily morning discipline of writing about it all, every day—rainy, cold, hot, dry. He *notices*. He is curious about what the things he notices might mean. See Tom's blog at http://www. thunderheadworks.com/.

Tom served on the Little Rock, Arkansas, development council and helped that group notice the uneven development in the city. Where to start? He and Wiley walked every foot of both ends of Main Street that cross over the Arkansas River, noticing all the broken links, the empty blocks—imagining what that part of the city might look like if it were filled with something interesting and valuable. At one point, he helped people notice the plywood over the broken windows of a former department store, depressing and ugly. "What if we made that plywood into a positive project?" he asked. He had noticed that other well-loved but dumpy communities had turned those walls into dreamscapes, asking residents to write on them, expressing their hopes, commitments, and dreams. People did, and the walls now spoke of the future, not an empty past. The dreams were almost more popular than the eventual development that regarded those blocks as valuable.

A Lovers' Quarrel

What drives Tom's curiosity? I think he loves the little hardscrabble town he lives in. What all those who love people and places view as sacred, blessed, honorable, worthy of praise and sacrifice are the practices, behaviors, and choices that lead to life, protect life, enhance life, extend life and spread life's blessings widely across the people. The Hebrew prophets always meant the whole public, never selected individuals, whenever they talked about "people." There can be lively dialogue between public health and faith because we are family— both optimistic about the future. We don't think God is done and we don't think science is done either. They are both worth pursuing together (even when some of us don't care about God and others don't care about science).

Anyone in a position to help people and networks move toward life must not stop talking about facts, analytics, determinants, vectors, patterns, and predictors. Get the data right and treat the analytic processes in as sacred a way as any priest would treat the sacraments. But we must *also* talk about our crazy love for the people—the public. And we must talk about why we continue to hope for a better world and simply won't quit hoping no matter what. You can take our money, put us in the dumpiest offices, and cut our staff. You can treat us as pitiful, not even as honorable as a primary care doctor, who in the hospital world is hardly on the map. We won't quit. Why? *Because we are in a lovers' quarrel with the whole public.*

If you are trying track the processes that are supposed to serve the public and cannot profess love for the public, it is urgent that you take your high-end analytical tools and move on down the street to do hedge fund manipulation, which is not played for life and death stakes. If you don't work from love, you're a danger to the public and the rest of us in the fields that hope for the public. Don't even tweet.

This is the time for those who just can't stop loving the messy, disappointing, ever-muddling gaggle of humans called "the public." We are in just the right work at just the right time. While others rant, we must speak out of love. We must bring our facts and our laptops, since we know that science is a friend of humans and shows us what we are capable of achieving. But we must always exercise our disciplines out of love, especially in public, especially *with* the public, especially about the things that advance the life of the public.

Generative Social Forms

Now that we've begun to see that the superabundance of life is already happening, we can begin to imagine how to work along with it. Life works better with a little help from humans humble enough to work on its terms. This is all about crafting generative social forms that help life find its structure. It is like working with concrete before it has set into the stone-like substance that can hold up aqueducts for a thousand years. That kind of concrete was so well formed that it has outlived all of its engineers, as well as all of the kings, popes, and generals since. It may outlive our fragile democracy, too. We talked about the fluid nature of modern reality back in our chapter about boundaries and why it is good that human social forms do not ever permanently set like concrete. While we might do with less viscosity than exists in our current reality, nobody—even the Caesars—would take the Roman Empire relationships above those still emerging through our current possibilities. We are not attempting to freeze and tame the fluid nature of emergent human possibilities, but to channel that energy through generative social forms that help life express its creative possibilities.

The one thing concrete and social forms have in common is that they are mostly mundane. Both demand careful attention to managing the weight and flow of gravity in the case of concrete and ever-present centrifugal fears that drive us apart and make us easy prey for fear. Theologians and anthropologists have filled libraries reflecting on that. More interesting to me is that it seems to be possible to hold both concrete and human potentials in forms long enough for good things to have a chance. Social relationships remain fluid, and this is our only hope in the face of our unprecedented challenges. Salk (1973) saw the discontinuities in human society as a positive break in patterns that would, if they continued, spell doom. He also envisioned that on the other side of each discontinuity was a period of social forms more adapted to the circumstances. This too would find another discontinuity as circumstances shifted and society would again adapt. Each adaptation on the other side of each discontinuity would need generative social forms to hold the energies of social life as the flow of life found its way across the many divides. That sounds a bit exhausting, but it's how we've made it so far, across many generations facing profound discontinuities. We have made it a long way; we should be able to navigate our continued passage.

Things that look adaptive are not necessarily generative; oppression is adaptive, too. Everything turns on one question: To whose benefit is the work directed? Dr. King died marching for sanitation workers because he saw that *all* work was sacred when done with a heart of service. All forms of work can serve life. There is no high and low work; only work that is generative and work that is degenerative.

Four Basic Social Forms

In any given challenge, generative agents need to work with four basic generative social forms: *projects, committees, limited domain collaborations,* and *poeisis.* The first two social forms—projects and committees—are familiar to you if you've made it through kindergarten and into institutional life. The third, "limited domain collaboration," is a more complex and open level of collaboration. *Poeisis* is a sustained highly generative relationship that you've probably experienced without having language to describe it, which we'll spend a whole chapter on later. So let me lay out the continuum before going into more detail about each of them.

All four forms have both social and technical characteristics that allow them to serve life better. The hierarchy is not about value or life-ness, just a differentiation in terms of functional forms. Generative agents need to be skilled in all four forms—and smart about which is most appropriate for a given situation. The greatest amount of time spent is on activities that appear mundane.

All generative work is social. It affects other humans and must take them into account as humans. You can't be generative all by yourself. There is no point in generating internal capacities that do not express themselves in social relationships with other human beings. The most mundane project—laying sidewalks comes to mind—has social implications. If you don't pave the places where people want to walk, your sidewalk project will be silly at best. All human work has technical aspects, too. Not even Dr. King could create magic when the microphone didn't work or the lunches didn't show up.

The basic generative social forms are for the moral purpose of protecting and advancing the well-being of the whole life of the whole world. Most of the time, the conscious energy of a team will be more focused on accomplishing goals that are near at hand and of immediate utility. But in no case is any person relieved of the moral obligation to work in a manner that is not harmful to generative potential. That would be degenerative. The surest way of contributing to the degeneration of life is to avoid thinking or talking about it. It is important to ask the question: Does the action my project or committee is contemplating add to the fear, friction, or disconnection of the social web it may affect? Sometimes it may be impossible to avoid these things. There are many complications in community and institutional life that inevitably involve some friction. Many divide groups for operational reasons. But is fear inevitable? I would argue that it always degenerates social trust and exacerbates social distance.

	Project	Committee	Limited Domain Collaboration	Poeisis
	Highly Technical	Normal Work	New Work	High Relationship
Relationality	Listen to take others into account, but just to work with as few as necessary hands on the plough.	Structure of power, but shared deliberation reflecting diverse interests.	Negotiated, fluid, uncertain, flat. Assumes partial investment that might expand.	High Trust Relationship; all in, often more than family, organization, or professional identity.
Precondition for Generative Dynamic	Enough trust and humility for the project to be useful and adapted.	Enough trust to convene and sustain dialogue to reach a decision.	Safe for vulnerability of association without presumption of full alliance.	Much greater shared language and logic. Goals far in the future.
Technical Focus	Do the work well. Good stewardship of time and money.	Decide and act on evidence to balance interests. Give clear permission or clarify the lines.	Craft *new* goals, bend and blend to do new things. Align assets beyond mere control, use life logic.	Protect the generative dynamic. Be smart *and* brave. Serve life of all, not just the core.
Biggest Danger	"Good work" is instrumental, not generative. Invasive, distracting, wasteful.	Unequal risk. Or unequal tolerance of risk. No courage so no action.	Too broad a domain stunts meaningful collaboration. Too narrow isn't worth the time.	Becomes a club or support group instead of action for the world.

Table 1. *Four Basic Social Forms and Function*

When we are speaking life and acting in the light of the causes of life, any social form is as deeply accountable as any single human to act in a moral—generative—manner. Anyone involved in any social form of activity must make choices that lead to life. The following sections describe each of the social forms in some detail.

Projects

The vast majority of work that helps the world inside, outside, and around human communities are *projects*. There are libraries filled with material on how to do this kind of work; you can become certified as an expert in *managing* a project by several associations of project experts. But at its root, a project is implementing or activating something that is already known to be doable. The project may be new in the particular situation, but it has been done somewhere else before. It does not need to be invented; it just needs to be done. Sometimes a single person can complete a project, if they have sufficient authority and resources. But often a team of people work on a project, all following (more or less) an idea or template that is trusted to be relevant to their situation. They simply do the work with craft and diligence.

You do not need to read a book about life to do a project. But it may help those doing the *doing* to see their seemingly mundane labor as serving the life of the team (by expressing agency) and organization (vitalizing the connections) and others in that type of work (enhancing coherence), as well as nurturing the seeds of hope by the practical witness of making something better. A project can be as simple as painting bike lanes onto a city street, or fixing a bad line of code in an electronic medical record so it gets the referral right. It might be getting the carpet in the sanctuary cleaned or all the members added to an email list.

Before you get all head-down into the doing, pause for just a second to consider the humanity of your project. Even the most technical projects can serve the life of the humans affected. And even mundane objective tasks can be degenerative, adding friction (which attacks connection), undermining dignity (which attacks coherence), adding to effort (which attacks agency), distracting from purpose (which attacks generativity), and confirming despair (which attacks hope). Someone asked where we might need excellence in the practice of FaithHealth. I told them to look for it anywhere there

FaithHealth

FaithHealth, a ministry of Wake Forest Baptist Medical Center, led by Rev. Dr. Gary Gunderson, improves health by getting people to the right door at the right time, ready to be treated, not alone. It is made up of dynamic partnerships between faith communities, health systems, and other providers focused on improving health. The partnerships combine the caring strengths of congregations, the clinical expertise of health providers, and a network of community resources. Partners are linked in a shared mission of healing.

FaithHealth staff, as well as volunteers from congregations and the community, offer health care ministries to anyone in their community who is in need. They provide support before, during, and after hospitalization. They make home visits, provide emotional and spiritual support, and help with meals, transportation, medications, and other needs. They also hold educational events on preventive health and wellness. Providers such as Wake Forest Baptist Health offer Liaisons, Supporters of Health, and Connectors, who help congregational and community volunteers provide care and ensure that peoples' needs are met during times of illness. They also provide congregations with educational resources aimed at improving health. FaithHealth trains volunteers in respecting patients' privacy, hospital visitation, care at the end of life, mental health care, home health care, and other topics. Staff and volunteers help patients after a hospital stay—everything from making sure their medicines are taken in the right dosages and at the right time to connecting them with resources that might help them pay utility bills or rent. Learn more at faithhealthnc.org is fear, friction, or disconnection in the institution. You can almost certainly see some of these from wherever you are reading this. Every one of the most obvious projects can add to those triple pathologies, or turn them toward qualities of life.

Sometimes an individual, fully responsible for a project, can turn that work toward the service of life by simply asking those on the receiving end how it might be possible to do so. How can I do this in a way that enhances connection, coherence, agency, generativity, and hope? How can I do this as an expression of my own creative freedom? You probably don't need to ask anyone for any more authority than you already have. Can you imagine asking whether you could do the project in a manner that would *add* fear, friction, or disconnection? Why not show just a bit of courage and give life a bit of help by shedding some light on the project?

Danger of Projects. The danger with projects is that they usually involve doing something technical that may or may not be generative. A body of work that could have nurtured qualities of life—especially the agency of those involved—can cripple precisely because of its instrumental success. The sidewalk was built; who cares about how? If a sidewalk is just one part of a more complex process of community nurturing, that same project can pull the energy out of the nuanced work of encouraging the connectedness of the neighbors, highlighting the meaning of the success and the agency of those involved. Whose hope was served by the success: the paving company or the neighbors who learned of their own potential? If the neighbors chose to have somebody else complete the sidewalk, that act of delegation might express their agency. If it was done just because officials didn't want to bother with the neighbors, it has the opposite effect. It's not the concrete that matters, but the minds and muscles of those walking on the sidewalk.

Another danger is that a project can magnify the perception of problems because most projects are initiated to fix something. I'm entirely in favor of having fewer problems, and yet I have served on any number of such projects. They are different from what I am inviting you to imagine here. Projects are usually designed around problems that someone thinks can be made to go away. And many bad things *can* be made to go away. Make them go away if you can! But don't confuse decreasing pathology with advancing life.

The classic danger of a project is that it can devolve down to the scale of the problem. The team evaluates its success or failure by whether the problem is smaller at the end of the project. You can measure a sidewalk by counting muddy feet or by noticing if people got to where they actually needed to go. A church project that began by imagining a new sanctuary for another generation to thrill with grace and hope can devolve into centrifugal arguments about the color of carpets and video screens. Hospitals that begin with visions of a healthy community often turn the project over to a technical group that devolves into distractions about hammering their electronic record systems.

Projects as Seeds. You have had the experience, I am sure, of having participated in a project that turned into something else. Because living humans serve on committees, sometimes life breaks out just where you would least expect it. The project designed around a pathology takes on a life of its own and catches the wind of the Spirit. (Technically, the wind of the Spirit catches it.) The project becomes a seed, the seed notices the damp living soil, remembers a dream of sunlight, and heads that way. Once a project finds life, there is no way to predict what will happen next. It will usually obliterate the problem that initiated the process, but the problem will no longer be the point. The group will talk differently among itself, about itself. Language of hope and generativity will find voice. This suggests greater risk, surprise, and understanding of what may be possible. A stone will have become a seed.

There is a very basic precondition for a project to be generative: Enough trust and transparency must be present so that the project resonates with the lives of those involved. This is especially true if they are understood to be recipients when they could just as easily be the agents of their own lives. A hawk has eyes tuned to the faint rustle in the grass far below; a human community is just as sensitive to being disrespected or violated, even, and perhaps especially, when the one doing the disrespecting is so oblivious they didn't even realize there was anything relational involved.

Projects can generate more than a concrete goal; they can nurture the preconditions for another dimension of social process—the oft-despised but endemic committee.

Committees

With the possible exception of email, most of us spend more of our work life in committees than in doing anything else. We all complain about how much time they take, but we're usually offended when left out for fear that a decision will be made that we don't like, or that someone will gain power that we wanted, or that some policy will take root that gets in our way. In organizations lacking trust, committees grow up where plain old projects would normally work just fine. Committees, like projects, rarely do the work of raw innovation. They usually have someone in charge and a clear hierarchy of influence among members. They could be, but rarely are, creative; they tend to perpetuate existing perspectives rather than open the windows for new ones. But no one mind holds all of even the most common amount of sense. And even the simplest organization contains people with different kinds of sense (some quite uncommon), not to mention experiences, skills, and relationships. Even if all you are doing is planning one more worship service, you often benefit from having a committee.

You do not need to read a book about life to run a committee. But life may want your committee to spend at least a few minutes pondering about whether it could be generative. Is life *entirely* a problem? What if the members thought even briefly of themselves as assets accountable to the life of the whole system and not just representatives of their special interests? Committees plan things, including new things. They create bonds of agreement among humans that are not entirely bound to the past. They can give permission and even encouragement. They need not only replicate and reinforce the old boundaries. John Wesley imagined a whole category of human structures that he called "means of grace." There has never been a religious leader more enamored by committees, which Wesley saw as the banks of a stream of living waters, giving form and direction to the flow. My father, a lifelong Methodist, believed that you could tell what a person believed by what committees he actually attended—rather than simply those to which he was privileged to be appointed!

It is common for committees to be criticized for how meetings are constructed or conducted. They are nearly always criticized for their fundamental lack of courage, and if not *that*, for crossing the lines into arrogance. What if the technical work of the committee were balanced by equal sensitivity to its relational qualities?

A committee is built for negotiation and deliberation, not the raw inspiration that might lead to flights of innovation. But...many committees are open to a brief "check-in" around the membership just to bring up any significant personal, family, or staff issues that should be made known to the body. The committee is composed of sentient mammals with human qualities. Any member of any committee can follow up with the rest of the members after the meeting through a carefully tuned note, a phone call, or a drop-by conversation. Sometimes you can open up space for humanity with a bit of coffee or home-baked cookies. This doesn't require a vote; if someone asks why you did it, just say that you appreciate how the committee is coming alive.

You can listen to the deliberations for clues of life, even in the most depressing agenda. While most committees "problematize" everything, you are free to ask, maybe even out loud, whether it would be helpful to flip the question into a life lens, asking: "Are there any signs of life amid the problem?" Of course there will be. Thinking this way might feel like a guilty pleasure, surely to be regarded as frivolous to some of the more somber committee members. But it will open a crack in the wall of problems. As Leonard Cohen (1992) notes in his song "Anthem," "There is a crack, a crack in everything/ That's how the light gets in." The whole point of a committee is to do the technical labor of making good decisions based on evidence that reflects shared interests. It doesn't have to be stupid in the process; it can look through the cracks in between those interests to see other evidence.

I once explained the expansive impact of the FaithHealth ground game like this: "It's not even smart; it's just not stupid. Stupid is ignoring the abundant assets and intelligence of our patients, families, and neighborhoods. We're not doing that. We may get all the way to smart someday, but in the meantime there is a huge advantage in simply not being stupid." A committee can do that with just a tiny bit of help. Life will appreciate it. But before you leap into the doing, pause just a second to consider two critical principles that help committees stay on the side of emergence and avoid degenerating into the opposite.

Principle One: Don't let work be more complex than necessary. In fact, because we already know so many things that could improve health substantially, we could achieve it with only a half a million projects and maybe 50,000 committees. This demonstrates a key principle of advancing life: Don't make things more complex than they need to be. What if every person, project, and committee operated at the edge of the authority they already have to do things they already know would improve life?

Principle Two: Don't let work be less complex than necessary. The second principle is harder. Projects sometimes really do need a committee to think more broadly with different perspectives. Sometimes what seems obviously useful is not. Sometimes the obvious way to do things doesn't take account of the latest science or better practices already known to an adjacent discipline. Sometimes a project is a hammer looking for a nail, when you actually need a screwdriver looking for a screw.

A committee can also presume that it is still competent even though the situation has changed in fundamental ways. Almost all hospital ethics committees are built to include everyone inside the hospital relevant to the ethical care of patients. But I know of few that are organized to include other individuals that health science now understands as critical to healthcare outcomes—the social drivers that lie *outside* the walls of the institution. A committee chaired by a doctor of medicine or bioethics is not remotely qualified to weigh the ethical dynamics of the full scope of the hospital's role in the social drivers affecting the lives of its patients. It needs community members with lived experience to add richness, texture, and intelligence to their discourse and problem-solving efforts.

Committees have a subtle precondition; their process has to rest on enough trust to convene and sustain dialogue to reach a decision. This is closely linked to the biggest danger: the lack of shared risk or unequal tolerance for risk. There is always a legitimate question about whose committee it is and whose process it serves. It is common for representatives of minority or vulnerable groups to be included on a committee, but not in sufficient numbers or powerful enough roles to make the process truly shared. They risk complicity, along with long-term loss of credibility.

A committee can be generative, if it is designed to be. The key test is whether the committee has the authority to do something unexpected or novel. If so, it is possible for a committee to nurture the ground for the next form of social process. At some point—you'll know it when you hit it—the process may tug at the edges of the imagination of the committee to the point where you begin to see the need for a social structure built for more unpredictable life outside the established organizational domain.

Limited Domain Collaboration

A limited domain collaboration (LDC) (Gunderson, 1997) looks *sort* of like a committee, but is in fact a whole different form of life. It is to a committee as a butterfly is to a larvae (and speak respectfully of the larvae, please!). An LDC is necessary in situations where a committee would not know how to act because something *new* or bigger needs to emerge. An LDC normally includes people and interests that transcend the normal operational boundaries and lines of authority in a community. Indeed, a limited domain collaboration often actively subverts old lines and patterns. It is built to find a way where there is no way. The obstacle may feel like a really big problem, but it is almost always a really big opportunity that transcends old problems. Limited domain collaborations are built especially for complex human communities.

Unlike projects and committees, which are well known by most people, LDCs may provide a new structure for your life work. This section will lay out in some detail how they emerge, take form, and enable change. All of these practices depend on a set of disciplines of abundance. These are systematic disciplines that hold us accountable to the life found where we have been taught to expect only problems. They are convened only in the presence of melting hopes. LDCs are built for life; especially the often surprising ways that life *does* find a way.

This life work is so much fun—even when it is laborious and tedious—that you'll find you want to discover other opportunities to work with the people who are finding life along with you. A committee is usually built around a *problem*; conversely, an LDC is usually built around an *opportunity*. Committees are shaped by the interests of their members; LDCs are shaped around stakeholders with an uncertain optimism about possibility. You could say that an LDC is explicitly designed to unleash the power of creative freedom in service of the life of a larger whole outside the boundaries of any existing committee.

All projects, committees, and LDCs are what John Wesley would have termed "means of grace." They rest on disciplines of abundance, but while projects and committees are usually built around some kind of problem, LDCs must always be built on a generative intellectual chassis. This begins with an absolute conviction about assets and abundance. If you can make a problem go away with a project or committee, you should do so. But if you sense there is something more tugging at your imagination, you'll need to be systematic about your approach to abundance. You may need to create a limited domain collaboration.

What an LDC Is Not. About ten years ago, the too-smart people at the Stanford Journal of Social Innovation looked at a few examples of what we might call limited domain collaborations and invented a back-of-the-envelope-level set of tactics that spread like kudzu through the world of institutional philanthropy. Called "collective impact," this theory depended on a "backbone" organization that would manage common metrics around a defined vision that could be advanced by aligning funds and resources (Kania & Kramer, 2011). You can imagine that I am not fond of any bit of that language and logic. But think for a minute about whom that might appeal to and why they might like it. Collective impact is perfect for people who are in a hurry to do something complex at community scale without all the bother of involving people on the streets most affected. It appeals to those under heavy pressure to move quickly (create impact). These are not by any means bad people—they simply have an attention span poorly suited to the reality of generative work.

The model of limited domain collaboration diverges most sharply from collective impact in its intention to grow beyond the boundaries of the control of the usual elites who tend to dominate the incremental improvement processes seen in most local communities. Ameliorating negative community phenomena is not likely to be generative unless it explicitly makes room for the causes of life of those usually left out of the room. A community is alive with capacities—visible as connections, coherence, and agency—relevant to generating a different future. But those capacities can only release expanded creative freedom if they are part of the process. Any process that makes any part of the community passive degenerates capacity even when it may be doing something that looks good. Saul Alinsky, the founder of modern community organizing, subscribed to this iron law: "Never do for someone what they can do for themselves." Breaking this law would do irreparable damage to the lives of those deprived of their own agency.

Collective impact has been extremely popular with funders and power structures who knew they were dealing with a level of community complexity that exceeded their traditional process of floating a problem in the air and then waiting for proposals worthy of funding to come streaming in. The "collective" part doing the impacting is often a very traditional center of power for whom acting "collectively" feels like a guilty thrill. It's getting away with something brave! Foundations are more competitive than cats in a pound, so for them to work together is no small advance. But it is not a big enough change to make any new impact. Few, if any, non-traditional powers or resources are allowed to play—certainly never an uncontrollable majority that might vote to do anything really different. It's comes down to just another committee exceeding its authority and funding projects that exceed its knowledge. Structures that are too simple or brittle stand in the way of complex opportunities.

A group of community change veterans led by Tom Wolff and Arthur T. Himmelman (2017), both widely acknowledged as experts in community and systems change, sharpened the critique in a way that sets a standard for limited domain collaboration. Collective impact, they noted, tends to largely ignore the need for justice; indeed it is a great tool for those who already have power, but is less suitable and more challenging for those with relatively little power who are working to improve the lives of people and their communities.

The core art of nurturing an LDC into life is the thoughtful, humble appreciation of the different kinds of vital logic of those finding ways to be together. The vital logic is the way people think about how their causes of life add up to a way of being in the world and staying alive in the process. It is dangerous to assume that you know a great deal about someone else's vital logic. So ask carefully: How is the group connected? How might those connections be more or less vital depending on how the LDC is defined and expressed? What is the coherence magnet at the heart of the group? How might that coherence be strengthened or weakened by participation in the LDC?

In the Mississippi Delta, very conservative and traditionally insular religious groups such as the Church of God in Christ found great energy through participation in the Congregational Health Network because it strengthened their own sense of being highly effective servants in the healing ministries. What are the existing capacities for action of the group? How does it already see its agency as being relevant to the emerging vision of the LDC? This is very easy to get wrong because of naive and outdated assumptions (e.g., churches have lots and lots of volunteers with nothing much to do) or dramatically underestimating power and energy. What are the hopes—especially those long unfulfilled—that might find new energy through an LDC? What hopes might make sense to other LDC members that violate the vision of one particular member? This kind of thoughtful, time-consuming dialogue is rarely valued at a table assembled with the traditional bait of old money, short-term grants, and the usual power representatives. It takes a lot of time, so don't expect it to happen unless life really needs it to do so.

When your vision includes multiple communities, maybe more than those contained in a single region, you need a very different kind of social structure than fits comfortably in the old model of elite tables. It has to be this way because of the inherent diversity of the collaborating partners. None of them really *needs* to participate and they all talk quite differently about their missions.

An LDC is defined by its limited space. If there is such a thing as bold humility, this is the time to bring it to bear. Include everything that is essential—and leave out everything that is not. This will test your humility, drawing you beyond comfort and dampening your pretensions.

A Case Study: The Undocumented. Although the LDC may—and usually does—expand from its initial limits, it needs some trustworthy boundaries in order to find a heartbeat at all. Take for example the need for identification for undocumented people, a situation that many communities face, including one I was involved with recently. We evoked unusual partnerships through assets mapping that brought together very different kinds of potential partners—legally, politically, ethically, and professionally (Cutts, Langdon, et al, 2016). Hospital administrations and sheriffs' departments are different. I don't carry a gun, for instance, or ever consider circumstances that might require shooting at someone. I don't even know how to think about that. Nor do most of the people I work with in the hospital setting. But we do count on the people wearing police uniforms to really think hard about shooting, as well as a lot of other highly nuanced issues that come with law enforcement. Both types of people are assets for life and have a chance to grow in the lives of the communities we share in common. Awkward as it may be, undocumented people make up a portion of the population a sheriff is committed to "serve and protect" within his or her county.

Undocumented people are almost by definition uninsured and we are legally prohibited from providing an ongoing continuum of care to them. But they are humans and, if they show up in our hospital emergency room, we are legally—as well as morally— obligated to provide the best of what current medicine has to offer. Other assets have similar sharp and distinctive identities and reasons for being inside, not outside, the limited focus that arises from the community process. These include the public health department, competing hospitals, the city police department (different mandate to the sheriff's department), and lawyers for all of these organizations and individuals, including the public defender's office. There are also community organizations such as churches and service groups, the Hispanic League, and many others.

Those outside the LDC can easily see the shape of its relationships and what they are formed around. Those inside can relax, certain that the parts of their identity that extend beyond these limits are not automatically sucked into the common space and presumed upon. The sheriff is expected to carry out laws. Churches, on the other hand, may well disobey some laws due to moral objections. The limited part of the limited domain recognizes the distinct responsibilities that each partner has. The level of trust in an LDC is as much about clarifying what it does *not* include as it is about the common work it *does*.

The nature of the limit is itself artful and subtle. Just as with a living cell, the nature of the cell wall depends on the life of the cell. What is it designed to let in and to keep out? How permeable is the membrane; how do new people and institutions come into the limited domain?

Growth at the Speed of Trust. Sometimes a limited domain expands, making the whole cell bigger; sometimes it divides, making more cells. The essential expands because of, not in spite of, bold humility.

Every discipline, field, and institution uses specialized language to describe the domain in which it claims competence and maybe even dominion. The sheriff is in charge of the jail, the pastor their pulpit, the surgeon their operating room. Here we move closer to the art of the LDC. Bill Foege, the epidemiologist who came up with the global strategy to eradicate smallpox, once told me that if you want to do something different, you have to call it something different. The new name should be so different that partners won't even recognize it. The new name is likely to emerge as the work finds life and form. The words "FaithActionID" (our partners from Greensboro who administer photo identification to the undocumented) pop up on my emails and I know what the subject is, even though I might have to take 10 minutes to explain it to an uninvolved colleague.

The most common way for professionals to define a working group is by the problem it addresses. Most people in institutional life are defined by the problems they expect to solve. Problem language comes naturally. It is easy, for instance, to define the many issues of undocumented people in this way. The basic logic of the limited domain collaboration can, in fact, serve problem orientation quite well. But this book is not about how to solve problems. It is not about how to problematize everything even more problematically. It is about how to speak—and then work with—life.

Keep reminding yourself that life is *not a problem*. Don't define your limited domain around the simplicity of a problem. The most inspiring goal that a problem offers is to make something disappear. Life doesn't want to disappear. It is a possibility that wants to express itself. There may be things in the way of life that are problematic. Gardens have weeds; institutions have unhelpful policies. But don't build the domain around the weeds. A farmer wants a crop, not merely a plot of pristine dirt. Call it a farm, which calls up images of fruit and bread, not just a patch of weed-free dirt.

The brilliant people at FaithAction, 30 miles down the road in Greensboro, North Carolina, built their identity around turning strangers into neighbors. When WFBMC's FaithHealth Division invited them into the heart of our limited domain collaboration focused on engaging the undocumented, they brought their culture and language with them. But not all of it; there were limits to the LDC in our little city that made our practice and language a bit different from theirs. In Greensboro, the city police were all in; in Winston-Salem, not so much. Any time we looked up, it seemed they were edging toward the door. Greensboro had the opposite problem. Their local hospital, born of faith like ours, was a reluctant observer while our whole movement was invited into being by the FaithHealth Division of the hospital. We met in our CEO's conference room. This defined the domain differently than it was defined in Greensboro, where it often met at the police headquarters or at the public health department. Defining a domain involves more than words; the physical space it inhabits also provides a valuable form of definition.

Sometimes turning from a project to an LDC—perhaps even to poeisis—begins with humor and playful humility. The ID drive in

Winston-Salem emerged from the assets-mapping process as well as the sand-in-the gears presented by the lack of an acceptable form of ID among the undocumented. This could have been understood as a problem that needed to go away—as it probably was by most. But many of those involved, such as Dave Franco (Leader of FaithAction), Francis Rivers (Chaplain Supervisor and Hispanic Liaison at Wake Forest), and Sheriff Bill Schatzman (Forsyth County sheriff), were grownups with heartbeats, so they brought their living spirits to the most mundane of meetings. Dave saw turning strangers into neighbors as his purpose in life. Francis was all about cracking open the room to allow for mercy. Bill took on the sacred labor to "protect and serve." Dozens of people in many roles brought their own deeper lives to the process, each gift humble in itself, but cumulatively creating a living stream capable of cutting rock.

At the first ID drive event, held at a Hispanic-owned mall, the undocumented lined up by the hundreds before dawn in hopes of nothing more than being known. It was an act of courage for them to simply show up in utter vulnerability. One of Sheriff Schatzman's officers brought a big bag of law enforcement bling for the children—not toy guns, but folding airplanes and soccer balls. Smiles broke out, then play. Some of the officers tried out their Spanish, inviting bilingual lawyers from the district attorney's office to find their natural (Spanish) voices, too. Today, many events later, a community has emerged from the original seed planted. The ID event has held its community together as the politics after the 2016 elections sharpened the divide between various factions and heightened real danger for people. Threats of expulsion have turned real, including the stunning case of a mother with a disabled child, who committed no crime other than being in this country. She took sanctuary at one of the participating churches. This has prompted other churches to step forward as well. This level of trust is only possible as the fruit of a collaboration that goes far beyond a project. This is not how projects work; it is how *life* works. In the next chapter, we turn to spend more time on the fourth and most delicious structure at the heart of how life works best: poesis or "work as delight."

STEP 5

Poeisis

Hopeful activity, no matter how productive, doesn't really seem like work. It often feels much more like play, in the creative sense of generating delight and surprise. This is the kind of activity that so stirs the soul that it needs a new name to capture its radically hopeful and realistic nature. It gives energy— seems to create it out of thin air. There is always laughter. I probed my friend Jim's imagination on this topic to find the right word, and after consulting a global collection of friends from Seattle to Africa, he suggested we talk about poiesis.

Poiesis is from the ancient Greek term ποιέω, "to make." It is the same root word from which we get "poetry," and was originally a verb, referring to the action that transforms and continues the world. Poiesis is not just technical production or creation in the romantic sense: poïetic work reconciles thought with matter and time, and the person with the world. Poiesis is, in short, what a great leader does with those he or she loves. It is helpful to think about past poïetic transformations one has already been part of and to see the fruit of one's life as far more than an assembly of technical constructions.

Jim taught me that Martin Heidegger refers to this kind of holy labor as a "bringing forth" (Gillespie, 1984), using this term in its widest senses. He explained poiesis as the blooming of the blossom, the coming-out of a butterfly from a cocoon, the plummeting of a waterfall when the snow begins to melt. The last two analogies underline Heidegger's example of a threshold occasion: a moment of ecstasis when something moves away from its standing as one thing to become another. It is the sprouting of an acorn that could be a great oak. No wonder our heart stirs when we grasp what is possible. And, oh, does the world so need just this kind of transformation.

Poeisis is the generative form with the least formal structure and what might appear to be a casual attitude about concrete goals. To take the concrete metaphor one step further, poeisis might be the place where the concrete is made, even before it takes its original recognizable fluid form. If a project is almost entirely an expression of the leading cause of life called agency, poeisis is almost entirely the expression of active coherence, which bubbles out of with generative hopefulness. It is like describing wind or another kind of energy, perhaps Spirit. Both have enormous power, but no structure at all. You can identify the pattern of energy in a force like this by what it does, but as soon as you try to contain it, the energy evaporates. You don't capture the wind, but you can design and set your sails by appreciation, experience, and wisdom about how it moves and how you might move with it.

You can see why poeisis and poetry have the same Greek root. Both are a bit maddening for those tuned to bullet point outlines and simple to-do lists. Out of deference to such individuals, let me try for some bullet points, so long as you don't take them too seriously.

Poeisis is a social form

- That emerges when a small group of people
- Who know each other
- Because of doing some kind of good work in the world
- That makes them think beyond their narrow tribe
- Or guild
- Or faith
- Or geography
- Or (this is really important) beyond the technical goals they began with
- And so find common curiosity
- About possible agency
- That raises up new (or renewed) hopes
- Often triggering new language needed to express
- New ideas.

Most of the most important things I've learned, done, and experienced have been in social structures with strong qualities of poeisis. Poeisis forms a bit like a hurricane, spinning off a social or conceptual desert in an undervalued bleak place—various countries in Africa or cities such as Memphis have always worked predictably as a metronome in my life. Poeisis spins in social space and emerges in what happens in between first a handful and then more people—usually edge kinds themselves, even if working in respectable institutions. If you need to imagine something fundamentally new, see if poeisis isn't what is trying to happen in your life.

Much of what we learned about the social patterns of boundary leaders (Chapter 2) applies to those drawn to poeisis. It attracts people who have strong enough egos to do what they want, but who for some reason—perhaps as in my case their mothers—have a strong inclination to want to do things that are good for others, especially those different from them. They have what might be called escape social velocity. Boundary leaders frequently experience themselves on the margins in a negative way. Sometimes they are so tuned to their marginality that they hardly notice the possible relationships emerging in the in-between places of poeisis. They may wander for years entirely consumed by their marginality. They are like vegetarians entirely focused on what they don't eat and hardly noticing the fruit trees thriving in their yard.

But...sometimes they do notice the life around them, including the other human beings trying to work on similar kinds of things. They've escaped the gravitational hold of their own core identity and group, and hopefully the escaping process has not left them so bruised that they are incapable of forming new trust relationships. They may be able to identify a new potential web of relationships emerging where the work of life is happening. You don't go from marginality to poeisis in one magical bound; it is an inherently complex process of life. But over time, something like a web of trust emerges that morphs into a web of transformation that, when sustained, becomes poeisis. It yields gossamer threads without brittle vulnerability.

Poeisis operates through strong but often foggy governance and outside the normal organizational calendar and budget constraints. Those involved tend to laugh more than seems entirely appropriate. The laughter is an expression of comfort and trust; also a signal of a high capacity to handle sensitive things (like money) more efficiently than a highly structured entity often does. Poeisis can convene, buy airplane tickets, reserve venues, and manage websites without ever needing its own normal functional institutional tools. It can borrow them because the whole of the members trust each other not to run away with the fruits of their common work.

I learned a lot about poeisis through the long and hugely productive journey of what became the Africa Religious Health Assets Program (ARHAP). When our group was first drawn to the ideas around religious health assets, we convened informally at The Carter Center and then found our way to Geneva at the invitation of Dr. Manoj Kurian of the World Council of Churches (WCC). There was no formal agreement or even clarity about what we were beginning to hope to achieve. The liveliest thread of dialogue was not around concrete ideas about "assets." Some participants were drawn like bees to the most obvious honey (which rhymes with money), or to exhaustively cataloguing all the hard stuff, just like an insurance agency or a police report might do. We let them do that while some of the rest of us followed a less obvious current of curiosity. Mary Baich, at that time serving as president of the Vesper Society, was no academic, but she had a sense that the gold in the dialogue was to be found in broader, more elusive ideas about assets. While we dithered, almost to despair, she drew up a simple conceptual map of the heart of our common energy. This was the hope that we could be more clear about what leaders had to work with to advance the health of the communities they love. Armed with this common hope, we found the energy, time, and plane tickets to meet again in Cape Town, South Africa, to live into a map that only emerged as we invented it.

Because of its raw creative potential, poeisis can influence and steer entire fields, even invent them. This also gives poeisis a dangerous quality that can turn inward and tribal, serving the worst possible social and political instincts. The untethered nature of poeisis is tested by one question—that of its ends: Is this generative for the whole world? There was no content or meaning around the phrase "religious health assets" until our group started living into the potential. We felt that we were on the edge of a "bounded field of unknowing," but the fact that we were there together made it safe and optimistic. We could—together—start to populate the field. One morning, Steve de Gruchy and Paul Germond, two brilliant ARHAP colleagues from South Africa and Losetho, envisioned a matrix that mapped religious health assets along lines running from the purely tangible (a clinic) to the purely intangible (trust). These also stretched from the most immediate (urgent clinical care) to the most distant (character formation). That's still pretty smart, even a dozen years and hundreds of pages down the road.

Generative phenomena may sometimes look subtle and slow compared to the dumb blunt weight of technical force and money. It doesn't take an army to be blunt and dumb. Any institutional structure can be those things if they overvalue the sheer weight of their "normal" activities. They can end life, but not form it; steal, but not create; crush, but not elevate. But sometimes even the most elite institutions can be humbled to the point where they know they need a whole new idea—something such as might come from an African poeisis.

A Case Study: HIV/AIDS. The World Health Organization (WHO) and its member national governments were totally overwhelmed by a tiny virus called HIV resulting in millions of mothers, brothers, and children living with a wickedly devastating disease called AIDS. The virus found its way along the silences and hypocrisies of power and gender exacerbated by colonial patterns of exploitation that mocked the traditional family structures of Africa. Dr. Ted Karpf was an early boundary leader drawn to the earliest breaking waves of the AIDS tsunami as the rector of the Episcopal Church of St. Thomas the Apostle in Dallas, Texas. I met him in the early years of The Carter

Center's interfaith health work as he was helping the CDC keep track of all the creative tools the communities were using to find a way toward mercy, even when most churches were ignorant and hostile toward the crisis. Years later, he was seconded by the Clinton administration to help the Archdiocese of Cape Town develop its regional response, and then he found his way to Geneva to tune the ear of the WHO to possible partnerships. Karpf understood the need for a whole new idea, and realized that Africa was a good place to find a group capable of thinking one up—maybe even two. He called me, wondering if WHO could trust us with some of their scarce cash to do the fundamental work on mapping religious health assets. "By the way," Ted said, "We'll need to do this for at least two countries." By then the seed of a poeisis was already sprouting. There was enough shared capacity in the group to earn that trust and immediately begin to do the work, beginning on the northern border of Zambia.

The story of ARHAP's early work has been masterfully told elsewhere in a book elegantly entitled, Beholden (Holman, 2015). Likewise, a significant literature has emerged around the enduring hub of Cape Town (Cochrane, Cutts, & Schmid, 2011). So I'll not repeat the narrative here, except for one aspect involving the most sacred of all qualities of poeisis: trust. Our first experiment in trying to map religious health assets took place in the battered industrial copper belt towns of Northern Zambia. Steve de Gruchy, Paul Germond, and Jim Cochrane had long relationships with each other and with former students who had built networks of trust in those communities. Steve had roughed out a model of participatory exercises based on rapid assessment of community development relevant to community-based health. We were all gathered in an old tourist hotel, drinking enough Zambian beer to fill the pool. Paul, about a gallon in, suggested a game where we'd each share a humiliating experience—his idea of great fun. I declined to participate, and the game went on without me—or so I thought. When Paul announced that it was my turn to share, I reminded him that I had already turned down the invitation to play. He declared this a "breach of trust." I had drunk a couple of quarts of beer myself by then, so without editing myself, I blurted out, "I don't need trust; I brought money!" Before I had even finished the sentence, Steve and Paul, moving quicker than caffeinated geckos, picked me up, chair and all, jogged down the concrete steps, and lofted me backward up into the air and then down with a mighty splash into the pool. Jim, in an act of solidarity, jumped in the pool, too—forgetting, until it was too late, that his paper airplane ticket home was still in his pocket. Nobody had to say the obvious: Never joke about trust. It's the most sacred thing—the thing that holds everything together.

Many of those involved in the generative labor that produced ARHAP as well as the Leading Causes of Life Initiative were formed in the tectonic pressures of apartheid and the vital movement that undermined it. Given the raw violent power of the South African government, it is an enduring surprise that it was brought down with lifeblood rather than bloodshed.

The Christian Institute of Southern Africa was as close to nothing as you can get in politics. It was led by a Methodist pastor, and its membership never amounted to more than a couple hundred oddly varied people of conflicting faith and political positions. They ate together near the train terminal where workers arrived and returned home to rigidly separated neighborhoods at the end of the day. They prayed, too, albeit in a mélange of voices rather than a chorus. They had little money and no guns—easy pickings for the powerful and little more than mosquitos on the back of a rhino.

In 1982 they had become annoying enough through their prayers and disobedience to be worth swatting down, so most of the leaders were "banned;" it was forbidden to meet with more than two people at a time or to communicate with each other. Jim Cochrane was a young man at the time, beneath swatting, so he was free to serve as a messenger bee in the now dispersed hive. The authorities did not quite understand how a hive could function disconnected. The Institute was, however, quite alive and quite able to overcome disconnection with its coherence and the ever-growing clarity of its message. The resistance alone was powerful evidence of its agency. Hope, rationally impossible in the shadow of Boer power, was stronger than mere political optimism. The group was pressed not down, but together, becoming ever more certain of its vital logic.

A community of poeisis thrived and formed natural vital relationships with other generative nodes in South Africa and around the world where others were drawn to hope. Both the Institute and the extended community had their physical connectedness disrupted, which made their lives awkward and dangerous. But they were still able to undermine the vital connections between the Boer church and the apartheid politic, the taproot of credibility for the whole political apparatus. A simple document meant almost as an internal memo lit the flame that burned away the bond holding apartheid together. Titled the Kairos document, this publication named apartheid as a sin (Beyerhaus, 1987), so vividly as to pierce the hard heart and allow life in. As life does, it surprised everyone—including those who talked the most about it—with the power to change the very climate in which political forms arise and then fall away. Not unlike the tendrils of the oak, the Institute helped crack a rock that could not have been broken through violence. That's how life works.

Today another weirdly virulent form of bad government in South Africa has arisen based on the power of stealing—captivated by money, just as blind as the previous one captivated by apartheid power. Further acts of generative labor—and poeisis—are desperately needed to bring this corruption down.

Built for generosity, generation, and generativity, poeisis does the hardest possible lifting in social and political relationships—it changes minds, strengthens hearts, finds the seeds of courage, and encourages valor. It finds a way, just like life always does.

I don't know how we could ever know, but I suspect that the early nomadic groups found their way out of Africa, across the Aleutians, and all the way to Patagonia because they had poeisis capacities. Other peripatetic bands crossed one ridge after another to the furthest reaches of what is now Scandinavia. Those small groups succeeded partly because of the huge advantage poeisis gives in a journey of radically dangerous uncertainty. The little groups navigated with generosity, not just suspicion; generation, not just acquisition; expansive generativity, not just violence. They were probably good with clubs and arrows. But there were plenty of other more violent and outrageous bipeds who you'd have likely placed your money on to succeed. Humans found a way because this little evolutionary offering had the advantage of poeisis.

Those early human bands, like our current ones, would also have needed to accomplish a huge array of other social tasks in order to raise generation after generation. Most of that more technical work probably looked a lot like Paleolithic versions of projects and committees. Many of us would have fitted right in. Early humans spent more time dodging big mammals and violent competitors than inventing philosophy. But the capacity to develop high levels of trust would have made them both smart and brave, forging deep bonds worth living for. It would explain a lot. The novelty of such a hypothesis is classic poeisis all by itself.

New Worlds Need New Words. Poeisis is often marked by the use of a new vocabulary. I learned the power of new words in Memphis, which is a city that desperately needed something new to happen. The timeline for this need dates back to slavery, upon which the cotton millions were amassed on plantations, to a massacre of freed blacks in 1866, to the assassination of Rev. Dr. Martin Luther King on our ground in 1968, and to the continued essential segregation of the school districts, even up until the early 2000s. The keys to unlocking the assets of Memphis were two new bits of language: the terms "strengths of congregations" and, of course, "leading causes of life." Two of my closest colleagues, Rev. Drs. Bobby Baker and Chris Bounds, read my book about congregations during their very last class in the divinity school program at Memphis Theological Seminary. Both were already pastors with successful careers in construction and civil engineering. When I showed up to take leadership of the spiritual care division in which they were serving as chaplains, they knew that I had a different way of thinking about congregations: I saw them as social structures with powerful generative capacities. I also thought they might be linked in ways that amplify their power into something much greater. The second idea, the leading causes of life, was just percolating when I arrived in Memphis. I was almost hesitant to talk much about the concept, fearing it might sound too chirpy for clergy working in the amputation capital (because of diabetes) of the South, a city that was also the crossroads in the national struggle between gangs—brown, black, and Aryan alike. The heroes of Memphis are those who invested their lives in a town they loved and could not look away from. Part of what gave their courage focus and direction was the new language that emerged out of the crucible of communities of poeisis in other tough places where other heroes were finding their way and inventing language to hold themselves together. A relationship that speaks of strengths invites dialogue about how those strengths might be expressed; maybe more is possible than you originally thought.

Words can be like smuggled hacksaw blades that a patient prisoner uses over time to escape captivity. Words can also break the legs of an infant collaboration before it begins to crawl. The most dangerous words for any young poeisis are those imported to comfort powerful observers. They can put barbed wire around the brain, stopping all thinking. The simple words "community benefit" are like this, imported from a legislative squabble aimed at getting non-profit hospitals to earn their (considerable) non-taxable privileges. Every hospital in America now has a committee focused on proving that their virtue meets their tax obligations (at least)—a very low bar indeed, given what's possible to imagine. And the word "benefit" invites the hospital to constantly exaggerate the positive influence it provides to the community while paying no serious attention to the "benefit" the surrounding community provides to it. Think how much smarter we'd be over time if we mapped the positive synergy found in community partnerships.

Don't frame a generative relationship—even a project(!)—around any word that limits it to some legal obligation or to the lowest common denominator level of commitment.

Protect the Beating Heart. Poeisis emerges from the carefully nurtured human spaces designed for real connection, vital meaning, real work, generativity, and hope beyond mere optimism. That kind of space is as precious as a living seed. Ask any mountain and it will tell you the power of the oak that cracks stone, not with its weighty trunk and mighty branches, but with nearly imperceptible tendrils finding their way through the soil into tiny cracks. These hold for a season, growing slightly, then in the winter the water drawn to the root freezes and expands the crack. That's how life works; we often wish it made a difference faster, but you can utterly bet your all on the certainty that it will indeed make a difference in its own time.

Occasionally, the work of poeisis is noticed by the powerful. They might be surprised at the things that turn out to be possible, rather like a timber company might be surprised to find that a second growth forest has matured in land long thought worthless. Sometimes the powerful will want what poeisis has produced. Generative work is easy to steal and impossible to defend since poeisis builds in totally the opposite direction. The powerful will mistake the fruits for the roots, stealing the apples and maybe lopping off a few branches, perhaps even planting a few apple seeds in the gravel. They are unlikely to notice the orchard, the long-tended soil, or the thoughtful adaptive pruning. In the meantime, the work of poeisis will go on and grow a whole new orchard (maybe peaches this time!).

Poeisis is sacred stuff and never wasted. Sometimes the structure becomes social compost out of which a new web and form emerges. This happens constantly in social and intellectual movements. Look at this metaphor just long enough to notice that it is vital precisely because fungus works in between other more highly structured forms of life (between an oak and a beech tree for instance). Compost can also be an artfully nurtured form, even a commercialized form (check it out on Amazon). In large scale generative phenomenon, highly visible social structures, such as the national coalitions I tend to find myself working with, often derive most of their intellectual energy from webs of trust that strengthen over many years. Like compost or, even more sacredly, loam. My most sacred relationships are like this. The vitality lies in rich, verdant interconnection and deeply grounded coherence. The "we" has from time to time expressed itself in things that look like committees or even grant-funded projects. Sometimes we have had "jobs." (I simply must put that word in quotes because the job is always somewhat accidental and, while appreciated, quite beside the point of poeisis.) Whatever task-oriented thing arises at any one time is well and good, but it is never the whole point.

For the most part, the generative form is this most basic poeisis. It thrives by the causes of life, capable of adaptive novelty because of its free imagination, trustworthy because it is always about the life of the whole, not about itself. That is what is sacred and vital and worth protecting. Life has, for several billion years in row, out-generated death. It will do so this year, too. You can bet your life on that.

Normal people don't think this way. So don't be normal.

The normal way of bringing people together to do something is to focus on the things they might fear that exceed their own capacity to mitigate or prevent. Turn toward life instead by simply listening carefully to whether there is any shared answer to one key question: What is the opposite of our fear? This is not the same question as asking what it might look like to eliminate fear. Any group of parents might be afraid to send their kids to a dangerous, poorly-led elementary school that is guaranteed to cause them to fall behind in preparation for high school, much less college. But what is the opposite of that? Anything relating to a complex transition in the lives of people you love is far more vital and alive than fear, no matter how well founded.

No parent wants something barely tolerable for their kid; they want something generative. And they want to experience themselves as participating in that generative process.

Let the powerful steal everything except the generative heart of poeisis. They can cut down the trees thinking they are what is most valuable. But, given rain, sun, and time, the land will grow a whole new forest. It is almost impossible to look anywhere and not see something that has been harvested, even pillaged, a number of times. You'll find seedlings sprouting in an abandoned Wal-Mart parking lot, entire forests growing on wasted, blasted, abandoned Appalachian land.

It only takes a lifetime, which is exactly what life has to work with.

Life at the Scale of Life

We've covered a lot of ground in the last few chapters. I hope you can see the most ancient and often annoying of social tools—projects and committees—with new eyes. You can also see them on a continuum that includes the more novel forms of limited domain collaborations and poeisis. Let's look at all four as tools that fit your hands as you do the work of life.

What if the opportunity you are trying to solve is really big, obviously beyond the reach of any project, committee, or even a significant collaboration? You'll need to use more than one kind of tool to build something bigger. My daughter is a pastry chef who creates cakes that defy the imagination. Some of them are massive works of art that happen to taste really good. The big ones are just like the little ones in that they rely on multiple skills and tools. But the big ones also rely on a greater level of carpentry to build the internal framework to hold the cake aloft, along with all the skills of design to translate imagination into batter, icing, and beauty. A large-scale movement is like that: 5% imagination, 70% baking, and 25% carpentry.

Case Study: 100 Million Healthier Lives

One of my favorite examples is a committee that looks like the committee to beat all committees. It is led by Dr. Soma Stout, a gentle pediatrician from India, raised in Phoenix, Arizona, and currently practicing medicine in Boston, Massachusetts. She is a humble master of the art of "committee-ness," nurturing the 100 Million Healthier Lives Campaign. This is a limited domain collaboration drawn together partly because of the trustworthiness that emanates from Soma and partly because she is flying under the flag of the Institute for Healthcare Improvement (IHI). It is an impossibly diverse group of people from healthcare, hospitals, public health, government, and academia, along with patient advocates and a few community organizers and policy wonks.

The 100 Million Healthier Lives Campaign is, in one sense, made up of hundreds of committees and a thousand projects defined and illuminated by the arts of "improvement science" for which the IHI is well known. It is exactly this respect for projects done well, committees doing well, and collaborations managed artfully to hold the tension of limited domains that makes the whole thing inspire confidence. The Campaign is made up of a critical mass of credible partners. Nobody involved has spare time, and everyone is part of other good and ambitious coalitions. Members are tantalized by how practical—doable—it should be to radically advance the pace of positive change through science and people of hope. What grownup could explain refusing to be on that committee?

One hundred million of anything is a big number. But we live in a

INSTITUTE FOR HEALTHCARE IMPROVEMENT (IHI)
IHI was officially founded in 1991, but its work began in the late 1980s as part of the National Demonstration Project on Quality Improvement in Health Care, led by Dr. Don Berwick and a group of visionary individuals committed to redesigning health care into a system without errors, waste, delay, and unsustainable costs. Since then, the IHI grown from an initial collection of grant-supported programs to a self-sustaining organization with worldwide influence. During its first decade, it focused on the identification and subsequent spread of best practices. This work reduced defects and errors in microsystems such as the emergency department or the intensive care unit. In its second decade, the IHI established a defining focus on innovation and the bold creation of new solutions to old problems. It reinvented multidimensional systems of care and began transforming entire systems. This work manifested in the renowned 100,000 Lives Campaign and 5 Million Lives Campaign, spreading best practice changes to thousands of US hospitals and creating a vibrant worldwide improvement community. Today the IHI is an influential force in health and health care improvement in the US and has a rapidly growing footprint in dozens of other nations, including Canada, England, Scotland, Denmark, Sweden, Singapore, Latin America, New Zealand, Ghana, Malawi, South Africa, the Middle East, and elsewhere. Learn more at http://www.ihi.org.

big world. Seventy million people say they go the church at least once a month, so we should be able to bump up their health simply by getting them to do things they've already committed to doing. These weekly churchgoers are within caring range of another 70 million of their neighbors. Even without worship, in the United States alone there are 100 million "worried well" whose health would improve if they stopped thinking obsessively about their own health and paid attention to someone else. If we think of the rest of the world (a good idea), the proper number is probably one (or even two) billion people capable of caring for others. While 100 million sounds like a huge goal, is well within the range of "OK, we'll do it." As long as "doing it" includes the full array of social tools appropriate to the different kinds of doing—projects, committees, and LDCs—it works. The scale is so big that it actually takes not one but several interwoven LDCs to contain all the social processes going on. It's a lot of life!

Dr. Stout has raised the art of collaboration to a very high level, while simultaneously maintaining a carefully nurtured culture of humility. It is as easy to underestimate generative strength as it is to overestimate the power of technical processes as projects and committees. Generative phenomena can look subtle and slow compared to the dumb blunt weight of technical force and money. But those things, because they are not generative, simply do not matter much to life. They can end but not give life, steal but not create, crush but not lift up. Life literally goes on without them, sometime without them even noticing. How we work with life is the most important thing to consider. It is the difference between capitulating to despair and finding the power in possibility.

STEP 6

What Matters Most

Crafting a generative social life means being accountable for what matters most. Because humans live by story, that means getting the story right. It means not losing the living thread. We are not held in the channels of life by instinct, but by the apparatus of narrative. In our modern institutional life, accountability often looks like data. But data doesn't form itself or interpret itself. Somebody has to imagine a story about how things work and then figure out what to measure that will illuminate that narrative. Data express a narrative, but they don't create it. When we speak of "accounting," we mean the process of giving accurate guidance to the work of life so we can follow its current as it bends and shifts across the landscape like the rivers we talked about early in this book. This is a kind of encouragement; the opposite of the scolding frequently associated with accounting. It strengthens our hearts, illuminates our vision, and guides our feet. It helps us look out for each other by getting the story right.

This is what we naturally want to do; we don't need to be compelled as if there were something we wanted to do more. But we do have to pay attention to our language and the tools we use for accountability, precisely so that we can help each other do what we most deeply desire—be agents for life. Joseph Campbell, the noted American mythologist, quoted Indian mystic Sri Ramakrishna, who said, "Do not seek illumination unless you seek it as a man whose hair is on fire seeks a pond" (1991, p. 202). Most academics do not act as if their hair is on fire; they rarely do more than paddle near the shores of possibilities. Who needs a pond?

For many years, academic medicine has thought that the pond was the great pool of knowledge they already had. They have tended to be pretty confident in their grasp of an ever-growing panoply of pathological "its": cancer(s), sickle cell anemia, diseases of the eyeball and toe, along with the astonishing varieties of "its" that collect in our arterial plumbing and lungs. And who could forget the terrifying varieties of viral "its"? Then we begin to think about the chemical it-things humans have invented that turn out to cause breakdowns and flare-ups that weaken and kill. I'm thinking tobacco, partly to avoid thinking about the thousands of industrial chemicals that also threaten our wellbeing.

Focusing on the pathological "its" creates a warrior mind tuned to threats and maladies and the impetus to fight them. We have built vast castles of learning designed to penetrate the veil of complex secrets that threaten us, all in the service of defending individuals against whatever it is most likely to kill them. If you are walking around over the age of 40, you've probably benefited from this kind of knowing in more ways than you might imagine.

Partly because of all this accumulated it knowledge, many "it" problems have shifted from being treated and fixed to becoming conditions that can be managed, often over a period of years, sometimes for the rest of one's life. That's good. The "its" of diabetes or sickle cell anemia don't go away like a broken arm; they can, however, be managed. The "it" takes place amid a phenomenon called a human life. Because you can't begin to apply all the sophisticated "it" knowledge without who knowledge.

This is difficult for an academic medical center (AMC) like mine, because a vast and expensive apparatus has been developed and justified on the basis that its research into "it" will save the world (or at least extend the lives of its people). The reality is that an AMC is an expensive way to provide evidence-based care compared to a integrated system of care that focuses purely on applying what is already known, especially to compliant "it-type" problems. Think about surgery and notice all the freestanding outpatient surgery centers in your town. They do the surgical procedures and leave the research to others.

You would think it would be a lot easier to learn about the life of our neighborhoods—the ones we are part of—than about a colony of microbes. There are, in fact, extraordinary springs of data that can tell us not just what zip codes to learn about, but the neighborhoods, streets, and homes that make up those areas. We can see who else we already know—members of our churches?—who might live just down the block and be more than ready to help teach us what we could do together.

At one point in Memphis we were working in a certain zip code because of the large number of our charity care patients who lived there. Chuck Utterback, the regional representative for CIGNA, attended one of our meetings and turned on the lights for us by pointing out that that same zip was also home to 8,970 of their members—

who we cared for—including 1,791 FedEx workers, 1,724 Memphis school employees, and 1,466 people who worked for the city or for the county government. Oh, and also 459 of our own employees! We not only had hundreds of church partners in hard places, but when we went looking for them, we found...us!

Honest Observation

The fact that the subject is us helps explain why there is a lot of nervousness when we start changing the fundamental rules of accountability from a focus on our fears to a focus on our lives. Think of Galileo, who turned the universe inside out (or right-side in, actually). He wasn't dangerous because of what he said about the sun and stars, but because of what that meant for powerful people who had tied their credibility to an obviously wrong idea.

This nearly got Galileo killed until he caved in pubic (but continued muttering in private) (Sobel, 2000). It was not the competing astronomers, with their ridiculously complicated explanations of how the universe only "appeared" to move, who considered him dangerous enough to kill. It was the religious authorities who had built their entire theological enterprise to support stability and privilege. Priests skimmed profits for their ritual role, providing theological justification to oil the gears. The big money, of course, went to the royalty and merchants who owned the gears that ground the corn (and the poor) into bread and meat.

Until technology emerged allowing a good look at the stars, astronomy was safe for the empire. But once the glass was ground, it was only a matter of time before an honest observer showed up and spoke aloud. If not Galileo, it would have been his daughter. Once the tools of observation found an honest observer, the coherence, connections, and agency of the old way frayed like decaying robes.

The shift from accounting for life instead of focusing on death is, by comparison, a more modest intellectual move, but it is still potentially threatening to the priests of the problem industry. Like the medieval church, the problem-solving industry serves the inertia of the political and merchant classes by offering up rituals that protect the status quo. They fuel the business of helping without creating any expectation of change. They actively undermine the idea that we could be accountable for accomplishing change. The most we can aspire to, they insist, is palliative care for the vulnerable. As in the medieval church, one can make a career serving incremental motions in the endlessly granular insistence on prospects for the poor being relatively static, capable of being changed only slightly.

Head Toward Life

You'd think it would be simple to head toward life, away from death. Any successful amoeba manages this. Dr. Gregory Fricchione, Associate Chief of Psychiatry at Massachusetts General Hospital, argues that this essential skill is baked into the process even of sub-cellular life and extends to supra-social networks (Fricchione, 2002). It turns out that humans are more easily confused than amoeba. Maybe we have too much on our minds, what with all the sapien sapien stuff going on. It turns out we need some help distinguishing the ways that lead to life from those that do not. I will leave it to another book to sort out the technicalities of constructing research tools that produce data and analytic models. This chapter speaks to the questions that guide how to help our work be accountable to life and for life. To what do we pay attention? What counts?

This kind of accounting heads in almost the opposite direction from the dominant models of evaluation, data modeling, and "decision-support." Almost, but not quite. You have only to walk away from your friends who are offering data designed to illuminate social problems and pathological phenomenon that lead to the therapy and behavior modification industries. Remember: life is not the problem; life is the answer to all the problems. People living in service to the problem industry are not likely to be of terrific help to your work of generativity. They may even be a distraction from life work, using up time, relationships, resources, cash, and privilege in doing work that is never quite the point. This sounds harsh and feels even worse when directed at individuals, because most of the people doing accounting and research in the helping fields are there for the very best of reasons; they want to help. I am part of a faculty filled with wonderful people who do this kind of work every day. Many have done so diligently for decades. They are decent, kind to their children, and accumulate global acclaim.

It's not the people that I take issue with; rather it is what they are told to count. They find their careers through relationships with scary, enduring, unsolvable problems. There are many problematic things that should go away—and I am grateful for those who make them disappear in exactly the same way I am grateful to the sanitation engineers who pick up my garbage and sort out the recycling. A city, however, does not live on what it consumes and disposes; it lives on what it generates. Build your life and the systems you depend on to guide you to life upon generative indicators. They will tell you which way to go.

Expect Surprise

The first step in forming a narrative is to build a story for surprise,

not confirmation. You are not trying to prove that you were smart before you knew anything, but that you were smart enough to discover
things that guide your work into an emerging generative flow. Dr. Nathan Wolfe, Chief Executive Officer of Global Viral Forecasting, has
said that viruses succeed—as do all forms of life—because of their
capacity for adaptive novelty (Wolfe, 2011). Almost any living system
lives because it—we—are more creative than the things trying to kill
us (mainly the gazillion trillions of viral and bacterial forms that view
us as meat). We live by novelty, discovered not one cell at a time or
one person at a time but as a social phenomenon. We live, in short,
by surprise. So make sure you build your learning system to notice
and elevate surprises.

In Memphis, I was recruited as a senior vice president to answer
one question: "What is faith for, in a faith-based healthcare system
in a really tough town?" I knew that the one thing Memphis has in
super-abundance is religion—which it needs because of its river city
capacity for sin. I was pretty sure that the faith that mattered to the
health of the million or so people within a couple hours of our hospitals who occasionally became patients was not the faith of the ten
or twelve thousand employees of the hospital. It was certainly not the
faith of the dozen or so chaplains. Those chaplains tended to focus
their time on 2% of the patients, those in hospital beds who were
on the edge of death. Those spending the night in our medical hotel
made up only about 20% of those sick enough to need a doctor but
healthy enough to walk in the door. So our faith professionals were
focusing on about 0.4% of our patient population. What about the
other 99.6%? Surprises about life were over there in the churches,
populating every street corner for dozens of miles into the delta.
Life's surprises lay waiting outside the door.

We had no idea how that worked. So we built a system to surprise ourselves. The first step was to organize ourselves around the faith that mattered most, which was the faith at the social scale, beginning with the place that social reality expresses itself by congregating. Nearly every hospital has a little data slot in its electronic medical record in which to record the patient's opinion about God, mainly to make sure we have the right voice to usher dying patients into death. We were organizing ourselves for life, so we wanted to know who our patients believed with. The social affiliation tells us who cares about a particular person, which is a lot more important than theology. Theological tribal identity (Adventist or Zoroastrian) reveals almost nothing useful. We wanted a specific group of people to work with. We want to be part of the tough journeys through life. We wanted the name and address of each patient's congregation.

Map the Connections—and Expect Surprise

Fortunately, at the very moment we were planting the seeds of what eventually became a network of hundreds of congregations, hospital technicians were creating the format for our new electronic medical record system, developed by the Cerner Corporation. They built it to be surprised, too. Long before we needed it, the system had space for the name of the congregation and a drop-down menu that made it relatively easy for admissions to insert the correct name into the patient record. The system was designed to ensure connection between the congregation and the patient by sending an electronic alert to the designated chaplain—and more importantly, the "navigator"—whose job it was to nurture the congregation's healing role. It was possible that when someone arrived at the hospital, they could be asked if they were part of a congregation that was part of the network. If they said yes, we could ask if they wanted their faith group to participate in this episode of care. This protected their privacy, which in Memphis is a legal requirement. It is also good common sense; you don't want your pastor to know everything.

The data system also served the coherence of the emerging living network by creating a large pool of data that could be examined in many ways to see what was actually going on with hundreds and then thousands of people over time. This offered up many surprises, some of which totally turned our heads around. I had widely, and with great confidence, predicted that the hospital would see a financial benefit by sponsoring the network as we built the caregiving capacities of the congregations. I thought that when we had enough congregations with enough training that some of our physicians would be a bit quicker to release patients for care at home. Even one day of hospital care saved by thousands of patients adds up to millions of dollars. I thought our network would help achieve this.

Surprise! It did help—a lot—but in the exact opposite way that I had imagined. Even before we had seen 500 patients through our network, and long before any educator could imagine, we had succeeded in building the competencies involved in caregiving. We were seeing substantial savings in the total charges for care, but zero changes in the lengths of stay that I had predicted. The data—built for surprise—allowed us to get smarter than we thought we'd need to be. Eventually, we realized that our connected patients were slightly more likely to show up a bit earlier, so more likely to go to a regular bed instead of the ICU. They were also slightly more likely to arrive somewhere other than the emergency room and more likely to be ready for treatment (they expected to be treated promptly and with respect because they had a membership card), and, most important, they were more likely to come with someone—they weren't alone. The first 473 people we saw brought savings of more than $4 million. Eventually, this surprise result became the core of our training, built around the mantra, "Right door, right time, ready to be treated, and not alone." It fits on a coffee cup. We also use this mantra for our work in North Carolina.

Trust is the Biggest Surprise

I'm embarrassed to type this, but the biggest surprise was that the engine of healing was trust, not medical skills. We should have expected that one. The surprising success of the covenant was almost 100% due to actions taken by congregations on behalf of their members and neighbors. They cared about more than the hospital. All of the factors that moved the data were expressions of actualized trust. As an African American man raised in Mississippi hill country, Bobby Baker, now Director of Faith and Community Partnerships at Methodist Le Bonheur Healthcare, knew that mistrust was the sand in every gear at every institution. So he quietly made sure that every design decision started with how that design would build or use trust. Once we saw the surprising fruits of that early trust, he had power to make that the law of the land, even if his boss was one of those most surprised.

The surprising data made heroes out of people we learned to see in whole new ways. The data made clear that they were teaching the system how to become connectable. We had little idea of exactly how 600 very different social structures called congregations were doing this powerfully positive work before we had taught them how to do it. We were certain they were accomplishing the goal in many different ways with many different roles. Some had parish nurses, but others had nurse guilds that were mainly trained to be helpful when someone "fell out" in the passion of overheated worship. Some congregations had medical teams with volunteer doctors, nurses, or EMTs. Most did not.

The distributed nature of the heroes heralded another surprise and raised new questions. Who needed the data? Who owned the data? Who was qualified to interpret the data? Who was most qualified to form the hypotheses to build the data collection strategy? Normally, "decision support" functions in a hospital are designed to fuel the evidence-based decision-making of the doctors and other professionals making the key decisions. Those systems are built almost entirely around diseases and condition-specific progressions of symptoms and outcomes. Even particular behaviors, emotions, and attitudes are mainly viewed as means to diagnose illness. Except for anxiety about social phenomenon, there is no room for the actual social realities of the patient. No room for encouragement or strengthening. This is not very helpful.

Honor True Power

About a year or so into the emergence of the network, the data drove another big surprise in the power dynamics between laypeople, clergy, and health professionals. The network rested on the power of the clergy and the hospital. But neither was actually moving the data. The ones doing the real work knew this and understood the life-and-death implications the data was showing. Bobby Baker and I came home one weekend from presenting at Johns Hopkins about how smart our network was. While we were gone, the female liaisons created the Liaison Council, which took control of the education, training, and learning functions of the network. We felt the way the early hindbrain must have felt when it found itself surrounded by a cortex.

Bobby and I knew power when we saw it and immediately honored the role of this group in setting the educational calendar, vetting new training curricula, as well as creating lively liaison training events that crossed all denominational and racial lines. The Council was not made up entirely of "grass roots" people, and it included individuals with clinical skills. They welcomed my wife and colleague, Dr. Teresa Cutts (TC), whom they trusted as a partner to model, analyze, and make transparent the constant feedback of real data.

The continuing data-driven surprises opened insights about the subtle ways in which race and class affect the delivery of what is often thought to be objective evidence-based medicine. In an act of courage, CEO Gary Shorb agreed for our system to participate as the only hospital in the entire South in a study on how race affected cardiac care in the emergency room (Robert Wood Johnson Foundation's Aligning Forces for Quality). We were relieved to learn that we were doing pretty good at providing the same level of care to both white and black people once a patient made it through our doors. But we were shocked to learn that black men and women were dying at twice the rate of white men on their way to the hospital. What the hell? Black chaplains were less surprised. They pointed us to a more useful question: "What could be causing this hell?" Who would even know where to begin?

We convened our liaisons, related to exactly those of our brothers and sisters who were dying prematurely. They knew, or at least suspected, that their people were so sure of being disrespected that they waited until the last possible second before calling for help. And they suspected that the same evidence-based care was not exactly tuned to the bodies of African Americans, thus resulting in the misuse of medications. Heart attacks express with subtle differences among races. The right care for a white person is not exactly the same as the right care for a black person. Quickly, we realized that we needed major changes in the educational materials developed for both families and medical providers.

Respect and Protect Your Allies

As the success of the network started to become visible in professional literature and government venues, including the White House, many researchers dearly wanted to get involved. But not every researcher comes with the humility to be a good partner in a distributed leadership model. A living organism develops a cell membrane that protects the integrity and vitality of its internal processes. We promised that no researcher would have access to our data without the permission of the Liaison Council. Protecting the boundaries of the liaison leaders created more than a bit of friction with the academics; nevertheless, it was worth the conflict.

Academics (my business card says I am one) build their credentials, reputations, promotions, careers, and often self-respect on the basis of their mastery of the specific tools used to gather and analyze whatever their particular discipline regards as "data." If you are one of those individuals, your life depends a great deal on access to experiences and communities that can be turned into data. Like sperm in search of an egg, researchers compete with each other, waggling their little academic credentials and hoping to find a way into a bounded pool of data with which they can have their way. The problem is that any collaboration depends on the integrity of the overall relationship, not just the priorities of the sperm. This often takes more time and subtlety to develop than fits the appetite of the eager academic.

Academics are not the only ones to exhibit limited patience with living systems. The powerful will frequently undervalue the generative engine, while hoping to take the fruits of intelligence, credibility, energy, and change that it produces. I can't count the number of "letters of recommendation" and "subcontracts" we have turned down that sought to wrap a cloying harness around the congregational networks to make them tame enough to serve another project. Usually the people asking for that relationship did so without cynicism. However, they were not humble enough to understand what made these avenues worth pursuing.

Prepare a Big Spreadsheet

There are other kinds of stakeholders who have the right to ask about their investment in a living project. While the largest number of CHN members worked for free (or for eternal rewards), the program did cost the hospital money and received help from other institutions, too. It is reasonable for them to ask if their investment was appropriate.

What kinds of data strengthen the trust of those charged with financial responsibilities? At some point, community partnerships will simply be the normal way care is provided over time, through government or private insurance. But right now, most of the financial justification comes from showing a reduction in costs. You will be asked to provide short-term data about the annual cost of "the program" and evidence demonstrating how it produces revenue (not likely) or reduces costs. The key is to build on the assumption that the most efficient possible system is one that manages to stay alive. But you have to see the whole system, not just its liver or its large intestine hard at work managing the waste. Don't be afraid of a financial spreadsheet;

just insist on one that is large enough to include the vital drivers, direct and indirect, that are moving the data. One year isn't enough data; track several year timeline trends. Make sure to provide costs and benefits of the system that includes the most vital partnerships, as well as indicators of the vitality of those partnerships on which the system depends.

When I came to North Carolina, it was partly because of the financial benefits that were produced by partnerships in Memphis. Some board members cared about more than finances, but many did not, or could not, care about anything but increases in revenue. I noticed that 30% of the roughly $60 million spent each year in charity care across hundreds of miles served by the medical center was concentrated in five small zip codes you could see off the top of the building and walk across in an hour. This cost was almost entirely the result of emergency room care for conditions that were easily predictable, given the poverty and racism that had kept those neighborhoods vulnerable for decades.

I promised to reduce that number using "proactive mercy," (Gunderson, Cutts, & Cochrane, 2015) and I needed something with which to be proactive. I suggested that about 4% of the projected total charity care would be about right. The CFO at the time, Ed Chadwick, found that amount by committing the payout of an internal foundation that had about $30 million. The board agreed to give me discretionary authority over the $1 million a year with the responsibility to report quarterly on three dynamic indicators: a) growth of partnerships, b) decrease in charity care in those five zip codes, and c) evidence that someone besides ourselves thought we were smart (peer review).

We developed a dashboard that included zip code-level demographics, including rates of poverty and population descriptions. We knew that most of the cost of care was actually fixed. Once you've built a hospital, you have to pay for it by assigning a minuscule percentage of its capital cost to every encounter. Saving a visit doesn't "un-spend" that money, so preventing a charity care visit doesn't actually help much until it sets a pattern that makes it logical to build a smaller emergency room the next time you think you need one. The second large category built into patient cost is the indirect variable cost—all the expert staff available in the emergency room whether you need them or not. This is very difficult to change. So the only cost that really changes—that can be saved and hopefully diverted to something more useful—is the direct variable cost. The actual cost of what a patient needs in an encounter. That is usually about 15 or 20% of the reported cost, which aggregates to the millions at zip code level. We built the dashboard so that it made visible what was most important to those providing the money. But we promised to succeed by our own rules of engagement, which focused most of our "ground game" on neighborhoods, not single patients.

Racism wears better clothes in Winston-Salem than it does in Memphis. The hospital didn't shoot Dr. King, but it did participate for decades in the ugly eugenics program that sterilized hundreds of poor and often black women because they were thought "feeble minded" or in possession of other defects (Begos, Deaver, Railey, et al., 2012). The last of those horrors was performed in 1973, which means that many sisters and aunts of these women are still alive as a living testimony to the untrustworthiness of the hospital bearing the label "Baptist." Many of the hospital staff from that era still live in the community, too. I knew it would take a while for even the most basic kinds of trust to be tested and found worthy, and for them to affect decisions that would result in patterns large enough to move the data. We predicted the data indicators would go up, stay there until trust was won, and go down steadily over time—years. We didn't know exactly what to expect.

It is hard for medical systems to see their neighborhoods. And it is even harder to imagine that these neighborhoods are alive. It is hard to recognize something you can't imagine. So even when the data did exactly as promised, the financial evidence was simply not accepted, mainly because it could not be attributed to this or that exact process, this or that exact "intervention." These are the things that both academics and administrators are trained to value. In Memphis, 600 congregations expressed their own intelligence and particular agency to affect change on a very large scale, but in terms of varied phenomena. This was also true in little Winston-Salem, where many different parts of a living system made choices supporting its most vulnerable people, making it more likely that they would show up for care at the right door, at right time, ready for treatment, and not alone. The aggregate data went down, starting in 2014, after it (predictably) went up the first year of 2013, as community members were testing whether our FaithHealth work would truly expand access to care or not (Cutts & Gunderson, 2017).

In North Carolina we did not have the same capacity to see the whole system because our data systems in terms of constructing early EMR platforms were already built. We did not have the same level of capacity to see our connected members and identify by them by their social affiliations. In Winston-Salem the level of congregational affiliation is less than half that of Memphis (surprise!), so our ground game, while social, was far more secular and diverse in terms of how we worked within the social body. We found that 90% of the poor we cared for were not part of a congregation at all (surprise!). And it turns out that the clergy and church people of North Carolina don't like to sign covenants as much as they do in Memphis (surprise!), so there was no easy way to keep track of which congregations were "in network." We could see the ones that were doing the things that mattered, but only half of them would sign anything called a "covenant." How can you attribute change to something you can't quantify?

Keep your eye on what matters most to the key stakeholders. Focus on what matters to them—aggregate cost by zip code—not on the process indicators they think are driving the changes. This requires thinking like a CEO, not one of the decision-support wonks who literally think inside the box. If you play down to the process drivers they understand, you will be driven down in both scale and calendar to the level of a micro-pilot. These are doomed to fail at demonstrating a process designed for a living social system.

Plan your work on what you know about life. Know that you'll need to account for the progress to those who may not understand it in the same way. Give them the data they deserve, but do not lose control of the process or you won't be able to keep your promises. You can't deliver on a life promise using somebody else's old tools that are not designed to work with living systems. If you make a life promise, use life tools. Otherwise, don't promise.

All you can really hope for is to promise results in such a way that you are responsible for their success. Ask for enough freedom to pursue the way of life that is necessary to produce that success using life logic. You can set reasonable landmarks—even quarterly ones, as long as they give you enough time for the life system to work, which normally is three to five years, depending on how much deadly mistrust you have to work through before life finds traction. They want success, which you can provide. But you can only provide it by betting your life on life—at the level of the system or at least the neighborhood.

The success of the Supporters of Health was quite a shock inside and outside the highly conservative systems of Wake Forest Baptist Health, so the news got around about the audacity and novelty...of trusting our own employees who actually lived in those neighborhoods and often had lived in them for decades. This didn't seem like an extraordinary idea to those employees, but it was radical to those with PhDs. Word was out that it might be safer than expected to do something different, at least if it involved helping poor people. Later, we learned that key leaders in the pharmacy department started their own version of "proactive mercy" based on the idea that they could provide home-based infusion for charity care patients instead of requiring them to present at the hospital. We already offered this as a concierge-type service to our well-insured patients, but the pharmacists knew that this was actually a great cost savings (at least it would have been if we hadn't had that vast and pesky mortgage on our $400 million cancer center to pay off). They tracked the data quietly, sort of like one pack of coyotes might shadow another to find dinner. Many of those patients, of course, were in our key zip codes, so they got credit for their strategy, but it also moved our aggregate accounting down, too.

The approach by FaithHealth triggered others to express their agency in ways that went beyond what we would have asked them to do. The pharmacy tactics were made possible by the cover of connection and following the same logic (coherence). Synergy causes the imagination to consider how to work closely with other parts of the system to generate more synergy. Hope becomes less abstract and delusional and more trustworthy, which calls out greater risk. Life creates its own next opportunity.

Root Life Assessment

The most important thing to account for accurately is success. Pay closest attention when life starts to move. It is common within institutions to do a "root cause analysis" (RCA) when something really bad happens. Everyone stops and gathers to understand what went wrong so it can be fixed. This is especially important when the failure was due to something that wasn't thought to be possible. How much more important to do a thorough examination of the unexpected emergence of life where it was not thought possible? Do an RLA (root life assessment) to accurately identify the vital life phenomena in play.

When life starts to happen, don't stop what you're doing, but don't miss the chance to accelerate and deepen the current of life by observing it closely, accounting for unexpected emergence, giving credit to every aspect that combines to nurture vital reality. How did the pharmacists come across the information that triggered their sense of possibility? How were they connected, and how did that connection spark their generativity? Where did they find courage to take such a risk? What are they hoping for now?

Enhancing the coherence of a living system is part of how that system finds its way, not just about how that system was smart enough to be an object for someone else's interventional expertise. A human system, let's say a neighborhood, is not a proving ground for anything. It is alive and will become more alive only by strengthening its sense of its own identity and the generative interconnections that, in turn, build their own agency capable of doing things unimagined. Don't rob the living system of its own dawning sense of agency.

Credit Where Credit is Due

Success can be crippled by attributing it to the wrong process. When the cost of unnecessary care declines in a neighborhood, a traditional evaluator will undermine the very process creating this success if they publicly credit some anonymous person working over in the hospital. The neighborhood as a whole and many of its members acting on their own achieved the results. The person over in the hospital (me) deserves a footnote on their annual review for being smart enough to think this might be possible. But if such a person takes all the credit, they will rob the living system of its own coherent sense of its capacity. This is an intellectual failure. Evaluation is a kind of power that affects the flow of resources. Intellectual failure turns its power toxic. It's not just a missed opportunity; it is actively negative.

Accurate evidence of a successful vital phenomenon expands at the speed of the trust won. Because it is somewhat unexpected—not merely the anticipated result of a problem-solving tactic—the evaluation is even more critical. Don't defeat yourself by narrowing the story to fit the old model in order to explain success. Help life continue by getting the story right.

Living systems find, create, test, discard, and thrive through synergies. Life causes life; the whole thing does the whole work, which is why it works at all. You can notice moments of time in which one or another cause is most evident, but you're watching an interplay, not a linear process. A simple walk through any forest will demonstrate the absurd lengths to which a tree will go to in order to get its leaves into the sunlight. Even if knocked to the ground, any old tree (not even the smartest one in the forest) will shoot up a branch to where the trunk should have gone. Utterly without pride, it just keeps on trying to find a way. The wild, endless creativity so easily observed in non-human life achieves a whole other level within and among human communities.

If there is success in a living system, it is about brains, not just boots, on the ground. Get that story right, especially in public. Get the individuals who are on the tough edges of the work onto the podium with the microphone in their hands. As the work in Winston-Salem began to be visible within academic circles, we were invited to give a closing plenary at a Washington, D.C., meeting of the Association of Academic Health Centers, a block from the White House. I spoke for two minutes with the closing 20 minutes going to Annika Archie, one of the initial Supporters of Health, who had been working as a housekeeper in the environmental services division. Following that virtual victory tour, our CEO Dr. John McConnell did one of his monthly executive video interviews, which normally would have been with me. Instead, he talked to me for five minutes and then went entirely off script as he encountered the raw vitality of Annika. A master communicator herself, she made the hospital the hero by allowing it to give her the chance to move into the community as an expression of its deep heart.

I tend to count keystrokes as work and undervalue the time spent in simple relationships. I am always amazed when I experience the power and protective effect of simply showing up and standing alongside someone who didn't expect my presence. The less expected the presence, the more powerful. It is common for politicians to show up at black churches when they want something. It is also common for officials, such as public health officers, to show up sometimes. From time to time, even a hospital executive might find reason to appear. But the church really doesn't expect them to stick around for the whole service, much less sing as if they knew the words. Go—and stay—when you have someone to thank. Doing so in front of those they value most is an especially powerful act. This may be thanking them for risking something valuable to a community process, perhaps on behalf of the undocumented or former prisoners or the mentally ill or the homeless. Thanking them in front of those they care about is way of strengthening them in their own generative work. Be sure to make them the hero of the story—not yourself—and to honor their creative intelligence, not just their role in helping you in your role.

Demonstrate Humble Leadership

There is no getting around the key role of leaders, but not in the way most people think. The key role is in how they play against expectations about their power to put the focus on others' power and generativity. They aren't merely being polite; they're aligning themselves with how life works. Where other CEOs love billboards touting their health systems as the source of miracles, Gary Shorb would say that the real "health system" in Memphis is the churches (hospitals are only faith-based treatment systems). Bobby Baker never misses a chance to elevate the intelligence of the liaison leadership council—but also the smallest congregation acting on behalf of one of its most vulnerable members. TC consistently uses hard data to make heroes and heroines of the caregivers who drive the data. "Look at what you are accomplishing!" She talks about their ever-surprising agency when she shares data in academic venues and at the White House.

Keep the focus on those doing the succeeding—those closest to where life is breaking out; the ensemble of energies and intelligences that live because all of the partners thrive in the abundance of new life. You will continue to feed the living flames of life by asking your partners constantly about how they are finding life. And you'll be surprised. Partners may talk about money, but more likely the focus will be on a complex stew of concepts, including trust, respect, and credibility. But whose trust do they value? You may value the trust of a local funder or the United Way; they may value more the distributed trust of clergy networks listening carefully for the voice of freedom, justice, or mercy. Take the time to listen carefully for the logic of how your partners understand their own vitality. And then tune your questions about "success" to the evidence of that vitality. You'll probably need to simply ask about it, but in ways that allow them safety to tell you the truth. You can ask, "Is your congregation stronger?" But you may have to unpack that a bit beyond "Are attendance and offerings up?" and "Are people volunteering for the care team and does that energy carry over to volunteering for the choir?" Try asking questions like these: "Are you finding yourself in new relationship with neighbors you didn't know before? Are members who work in public services like sanitation, law enforcement, teaching, or city government feeling more valued?" If you show that you have a broader understanding of the vital nature of congregational life, you'll open up space for a more life-encouraging answer.

Until a leader sees a pattern, they are powerless to do anything but react out of fantasy or fear. Their action is arbitrary or random. Even success is dangerous in these situations because it results from action that is disconnected from reality. Good data helps sensitive leaders find the true patterns in stories. Good narratives help sensitive leaders find the true story in the data.

Speak the Right Language

A senior colleague once came to me with the happy news that she had been approved to include me in her annual goals for the next year. "We all love what you do," she said, "but have no idea what it is. The problem is that we all speak German and you speak Greek. I'm going to learn to translate you so we can help more." "Ah," I replied, "it is much worse than that. I don't speak Greek; I speak Sesotho! And the subject is not hospital operations, but bophelo!"

Sesotho is the language of the people living in the high mountains of Lesotho. In Sesotho, there is no way to talk about health without implying the spiritual dimension. Likewise, there is no word in which you can speak about the Spirit and not imply the health of everything—the body, the family, the neighbors, the streams, and the grazing cattle. The language simply does not permit the separation of the concept we are struggling to connect in English. Closest to the word shalom, bophelo is the best word to use in speaking of life. The influence of this word is why there is no space in FaithHealth, the name of our division. My title is Vice President for FaithHealth, not faith and health. The operational plans, budgets, job descriptions, fieldwork, and "ground game" only make sense in light of that unity. And all of our individual tasks and doing-of-good is measured against it. That is how life is organized—and how the work that nurtures life is to be evaluated.

I do speak a little German. Also public health, which is a dialect. I have carried a business card as faculty, now professor, of public health for many years now. I find the sciences, if broadly and artfully employed, to be the friend of human flourishing. But it is good advice to refuse to allow them to drive drunk on their own wine. Hold them accountable to their most noble virtues—uncertainty and curiosity. When the sciences—social, physical, biological, chemical, or physical—devolve into tools for proving this or that, they lose their own love of coherence and sacrifice their generative agency in service of creative imagination for the thin gruel of proof. I see this even in my colleagues in public health, that mélange of sciences dedicated to advancing the health of the ragged gaggle of people called the public.

Using the right language extends to being generous, generative, and accurate with titles, honors, and relationships. Accurate titles and names can be awkward to give, but focus attention on the novelty of the role. Something different is going on, which is exactly what you want to protect. When Supporters of Health began, I almost accidentally offered the group the chance to name this new role. We didn't want it to just be a community health worker or clinical extension. I had in mind "agent of healing" or even more bizarre "agent of the reconciliation." They chose "Supporter of Health," which I hated at the time, but eventually came to see as profoundly accurate. Language like this makes sense if one is trying to advance the health of the whole population, but it can sound funny to those slowly working their way out their deductive, linear, operational cave.

Identify the Hero (It's Not You)

Whatever you do, don't make yourself the hero of someone else's story. Give headlines to those who need them most. Protect the creative imagination of those most likely to be vulnerable. Also be aware that the quickest way to make someone even more vulnerable is to make them a hero in a story that competes with those they need to cooperate with in order to survive. A hospital up the road from us has a bit of a proud spirit and is loathe to think they could learn anything from us. They see FaithHealth as a very simple set of tasks that they need no assistance to achieve. How hard could it be? After observing the model from afar and sitting through a single conference call, a senior executive took on responsibility for beginning their own program.

One minor challenge was that one of their smaller hospitals in one of the very most difficult mountain counties was already using our model and showing pretty amazing outcomes. The heroes of the story were being overlooked, undervalued, and actually facing reduced support. It would certainly not have helped for them to be seen as the minions—even successful ones—of a competitor down the hill. The local lead was one of our FaithHealth Fellows with two extraordinary "connectors" who had become deeply woven into the fabric of the mountain county. The connectors—working officially one day a week each—had provided more than 10,000 miles of healthcare transportation over just one year to the hospital patients who would almost certainly have failed to attend their appointments, had their conditions managed, and achieved healing. We gave Phillip Long, their FaithHealth Fellow, the microphone at a state summit on transitions in care, and made sure the story got into the local newspaper. And we did a careful case study of the work of the connectors to document the clinical and financial implications of their work—finally explaining those outcomes in the generative logic of FaithHealth.

It was not an accident that Phillip had external funds with which to finance the connectors initially. TC wrote the grant that way so that a competitor's staff could achieve outcomes for which they would receive credit. Giving things away, including cash and credit, builds the credibility of the generative community, so everyone gains, including us. We had to argue with our own fundraising staff to do the grant this way, of course. They couldn't understand why we would give away money we'd earned based on what they understood to be our prestige so that a competitor would also gain prestige. I had just barely enough institutional power to push my way through. In fact, fundraisers get credit for every dime they raise, so they don't really care all that much where the money goes. I gave them credit, too.

This kind of generative phenomenon strengthens the whole network, but you have to work on getting the story right or the story will dumb right back to making the hero the one who would normally be the hero. In my context, that hero would be me, the senior person with the impressive business card. But the hero is the one on the edges of the generative phenomenon. The hero in this story is, in fact, Phillip and his amazing two connectors and dozens of volunteers in McDowell County, North Carolina. The generative whole has to be constantly reinforced with language that turns the attention and appreciation to those doing the work. Under pressure the old story will come right back. You have to be constantly telling—and creating—the new one.

STEP 7

Chaos Fights Back

I tend to live on the happy side, which is what you might expect from a person writing a book about life while many see the planet boiling with vitriol and hot air. The youngest child of five in a white middle-class professional family living in the 'burbs, I grew up with things just sort of working out OK for me. My mom was unusually cheerful, which gives me a skewed view of reality that works for me. Optimism tends to be self-fulfilling—and annoying to those with more normal experiences of life.

In 2005 I moved to Memphis and participated in a remarkable phenomenon of spirit and raw humanity that released hopeful and healing energies into thousands of lives. This wasn't surprising to just me, a white liberal from Atlanta. It surprised some of the most grounded pastors in the African American churches who had lived in the wash of the Spirit amid the raw and bloody edges of racism in the tortured mud of the delta, which extended up and onto the rich bluffs of Memphis. They had good mothers just like mine, but were raised with warnings born of love. It's a bitter land for the poor.

The work in Memphis found traction, showed success, and attracted local, regional, and national regard. But one day one of my chaplains, Chris Bounds, came into my office, closed the door, and said, "This is just Chris and Gary." I knew it was serious because he was a man humble before God, but one who looked every human in the eye. In his kind voice, he told me that I was unequipped to live in Memphis because I had no understanding of evil. "Brother, you may not believe in Satan, but you have to have some way to see that evil is alive and real in the world or you are utterly defenseless with your happy optimism. You're gonna get us all killed."

The story of human history is not just about progress. The brokenness in the world that breaks our hearts is not just a list of things needing to be fixed. The ugly, deadly, and demented edges that hurt the weak and crush the hopes of the poor are not just things that haven't quite worked out yet. It is not just that chaos has not quite yet been tamed and ordered.

Chaos fights back.

Life does not just move into empty space. There is no empty space in our little round planet.

It is life against death; life against the forces of disconnection, incoherence, powerlessness, entropy, and fear. Forces of generation fight with those of active degeneration. It is life for the whole contesting with those who would graze on the hopes and the bodies of the poor. It is life against death, but it's a fair fight—all that a grownup could hope for.

I am still sorting through Chris's counsel about Satan. I have seen the face of chaos and know its power to derail, distract, and confuse the hearts and spirits of any and all of us. There is a reason that one of the names Chris uses for Satan is "deceiver." We are easy to confuse and often confuse ourselves. Several million really smart people are at this very moment deploying carefully tuned messages to deceive you into worrying about something in your life that could be fixed by handing them money, time, or votes. We end up with a lot of plastic, pills, and distractions so unhelpful that we are even easier prey for the next anxiety. We are deceivable and ultimately capable of forgetting the most important things that give us joy, meaning, and life. I'm not sure we need an actual devil to account for this pervasive confusion. The same humans getting us to worry ourselves to distraction are themselves worried. (I need another hotel! Maybe an island?)

I am closer to Salk than Satan on this; our great capacity for novel adaptation means we need to learn wisdom in continually new circumstances. This is why a discontinuity is a true break that we can only navigate by the lights of life. We are anxious because things are fluid and changing. We live in great vulnerability, easily convinced to look backward into chaos when life lies ahead.

The powers of chaos—however you understand them—are vulnerable themselves because they believe in their own flawed power and underestimate the strength of generative phenomenon. Life doesn't have to beat death, it only has to out-generate it, generation after generation.

You don't sustain life as you would something that is not alive. We are tempted to trust the brittle strategies of boundaries, bricks, and dumb power, but there is no real protection for

things because they are not alive and cannot adapt. Things—
and those who trust in things—always give way to entropy and
change. If you're a mountain, you should pay attention to tectonic subduction. Every empire and royal tribe has tried to sustain their follies on piles of others' bones until theirs also join
the pile. Some were prescient enough to write their names in
hard stone, so we can at least read their names later on. They
no doubt hoped for more. Meanwhile, the most fragile of all relationships, such as that of an itinerant carpenter and His odd
gaggle of the people He called friends, lives across millennia.
The community of spirit somehow holds the energy of generative freedom and moves toward life. That gaggle itself proved
easily deceived by the embrace of empire and vapid politics, but
still remembered—often in the nick of time—that in the beginning and in every new beginning is the word of life.

As chaos does, and ever will, fight back, our task is to protect
the possibility of the idea of life.

Look Out for Each Other

The first task of a generative agent is to nurture, strengthen,
and sometimes protect others open to the emergence of life. If
you have any power, privilege, resources, capacities, or a voice,
your first job is to invest these things in protecting those who
have less of them. They are already risking what they do have in
the same generative hope you carry. I am talking about the very
practical and tactical tasks of taking care of those exposed in the
work of life.

Generative agents must protect the generative social nodes,
out of which will come the lasting qualities of creative adapt-

ability. This is a contested work, since there is a lot of competing energy going into protecting those dedicated to ameliorating the conditions of the past. The problem solvers will become only more urgent in their claims on resources and privileges as the problems of the past become worse, making it harder to see alternatives. Ironically, the only way to solve those problems on a large scale is to give over to a whole new way of understanding the dynamics within the discontinuity. Life works better than any pathology-based approach. Indeed, life is almost always the only thing that works, even when proponents of the old lenses assign credit elsewhere.

Those living into their roles as generative agents will constantly be vulnerable among those of the dominant problem-solving model in their organization. Generativity looks soft compared to the hard edge of a problem, even if the problem-solvers often have little to show for their efforts. They are following the expected playbook (they often actually have a thing called a playbook!). And we should be grateful—I repeat, grateful—that when we have a problem, there are problem-solvers around who know just what to do. The challenge of working for or with an organization built on problems is that it is difficult to defend resources—sometimes even a job—when turning from pathology to generativity. The generative arts simply look indirect and the successes more difficult to attribute accurately.

It is important for those living within and counting on and working through generative networks to protect each other. Look out for the individuals most exposed. This may look different depending on what they are exposed to. I work in an organization enthralled with the problem-solving spirit. We even have a banner in front of which about a hundred people gather every morning in a "safety huddle." The banner proclaims that we are "obsessed with failure," which could hardly be stranger for a group focused on health. The point is that anyone in the organization who shows creative imagination and generous novelty is swimming in cold waters going against the current. In these waters our little FaithHealth division got away with a very bold body of work dedicated to proactive mercy, which we've mentioned earlier. Our success—and the fact we didn't get killed for it—encouraged others in more normal parts of the organization who had the identical spirit, but less freedom to express it—the pharmacy, as described in a previous chapter.

On the face of it, you might not really want your pharmacist thinking like a creative risk-taker. Just give me the pill the doctor prescribed. (Except when it is the wrong pill due to a conflict with another pill the doctor might not have thought about. Oh, and check the handwriting or typing to make sure the pill and dosage makes sense. And while you're at it, check to see if the pill prescribed is affordable to the patient and thus has a chance to be used.) There's more to think about than you might think, because pharmacists are in the middle of a number of highly complex human processes.

In the example shared earlier, the pharmacy department (one or two particular members, actually) noticed the creative imagination being expressed over on the FaithHealth side of the hospital and saw a big opportunity to do the right thing at the right time in another way. They just sort of...did the right thing in a way that was not specifically prohibited, but not explicitly ordained either. In short, they gave away infusion medicine to the poor in their homes, something we do for rich and well-insured people every day with very specific medical protocols. The pharmacists carefully documented (as pharmacists do) powerful evidence of the effectiveness and cost-saving benefits of their proactive mercy. But they took a real risk, were actually vulnerable, and could have been hurt, even if only by seeming suspect for having spent a bit too much time thinking about poor people who are, well, poor. That might not sound especially brave, but it was.

I had no direct organizational power with which to protect these individuals. They didn't work for me. But I was careful to make sure the Board of Directors' committee I manage heard about this as evidence of how widely the spirit of "proactive mercy" was expressing itself within the organization they were responsible for. We shared pharmacy data—and the story of their creative professionalism—which made them heroes among the governance. This was real protection as they emerged from the arcane shadows deep in the bowels of the risk-averse organization into the sunlight of "community benefit." And we made sure that the story included the hard-edged financial results the board is responsible for caring about, as well as the warm and touching narrative of vulnerable people receiving much better care than usual. To do one without the other keeps the "proactive mercy" over in the nice-but-optional category, which would have endangered the pharmacists and everyone else associated with this purely optional mission. If I did not have the power of planning the board committee agenda, I might have done pretty much the same thing by publishing an article about it in our division newsletter and maybe gotten the medical center news people to publish a story, too. I could have also written an op-ed in the city newspaper, making sure the CEO (and board) saw it. The point is, when someone does what you'd want them to do—use some of your means of protection to help them.

Last chapter we touched on how important it is to protect those doing generative work by getting the story right. Give the generative agents credit, especially when the life process provides some gain valuable to old institutions. The organization may worry about how to decrease unnecessary admissions, decrease jail recidivism, improve recovery from drug dependency, or lower adolescent suicides. Life processes will do all these things, but in ways that are strikingly different from how these goals are usually approached by problem-solvers. If you let the story of the success be told through the narrative framework of those traditional models, it will not protect the generative agents, even if they are mentioned in a positive light. They will still be role-players in the wrong narrative, getting credit for acting out traditional behaviors understood to be effective according to the old ways. This is where you have to get the story right about the logic and approach—but also make sure to include the success indicators that would normally be expected to be produced in the old way. Give credit to the generative process and to the actors producing success according to the new way.

When something works in a new way, make sure you give credit both to those showing courage and to how they showed courage. Many organizations with a long history carry very old stories of obedience to whoever (temporarily) holds a role of power, such as mine. In this sense, power is like one of those dangerous things that deceives us and distracts from what really works. In highly fluid times such as ours, it is dangerous to expect anyone at the center to be smart enough to find the way by themselves. Learning networks are "smart on the edges." And they will get smarter and stronger as we set those edges free to do the next right thing. That's easy for me to say—I'm the one in power. What is important is to make sure that when someone on the edges shows agency (along with connection, coherence, generativity, and hope)—that they are encouraged.

Most leaders want to know about every little thing, as if they could possibly be smart enough to direct it all. You may be able to do that in a dumb, slow system, but you can't in a smart, adaptive one. I want life, so I want surprises. I'm happy to give up the apparent efficiencies of control for the real efficiencies of adaptive systems.

Don't forget to honor powerful people when they do the right thing. Honor the board and financial department for their careful stewardship of money. We might disagree over how large a margin a non-profit hospital needs, but not over whether it should be as utterly efficient as possible. The things that lead to efficiency are honorable labor, just as are acts of charity. Both are forms of stewardship. I'm glad that our generative community approaches are efficient and cost-effective. I'm happy for that to be part of our story. I never ask for any special privileges or slack because of the "spiritual" nature of my work, even though most boards and senior leaders would give some if there were enough margin to provide some slack. What protects the process for all the spinning, popping, emerging, and surprising is constantly looking for and accurately capturing the story of how the process advances goals valuable to the stakeholders, some of whom may not understand or even appreciate the way the work is moving. The key to this is understanding what those stakeholders actually want and value.

The challenge is to focus on life in the tough places, lean years, and most difficult challenges. It's not what you talk about after the work is done; it is the work and the way it works. The only way to protect the generative community within and around the institution is to constantly build a reputation along those lines. When times are worst, you want people to think of your generative work—"Those folks (like life) find a way." Don't be a genius; be someone who lives with deep appreciation in a community of people smart about life.

What the Past Gets Wrong

The past deceives us by asking us not to take the possibilities of our one life seriously. In anxious times, we listen too carefully to all that the past teaches us about what has not worked. The past hides the most important things in plain sight, including the simple fact that history doesn't repeat. It happened, but it isn't destiny. It circles, as does the hawk above me as I type this; once, twice, then another six times, but never in quite exactly the same way. Finally, having seen enough, it lets the breeze over the ridge carry it down and away into another life. History is not a circle but a spiral, never quite repeating.

The challenge for us short-lived ones is that some life lessons take more than one lifetime to clarify. This is especially true for the bad things. Wrong can triumph for a long, long time, far beyond what you'd think possible. Bad people often get away with things for pretty much their entire lifetimes. Sometime their kids pick right up where the parents left off and they get away with bad things, too. But Dr. King wasn't delusional when he saw the arc of history bending toward justice.

Sometimes it takes more than one lifetime for even the most obvious good things to mature. All my life it seemed obvious that the sun was giving us plenty of energy every day, beyond any possible amount that could ever be needed. That could be enough for billions of trees to grow and trillions of plankton to feed all the fish in the swirling oceans. Or surely enough to warm our little human houses and to allow us to move around without bothering the horses. It was always out of reach, the iconic tree-huggers' folly. Until in a blink it wasn't. And in another blink the Peabody coal train was the folly. China—no country of tree huggers—cancelled a hundred coal-burning power plants and started covering desert sands with silicon wafers. Some dreams long deferred are just waiting for the converse to emerge.

This is not just true of technology, which is created by small groups of people acting ahead of what seems possible at any given time. In recent decades millions of wholly new organizations have been invented for the purpose of doing something new, usually intended for some sort of good. These groups compete with each other in some sense, always prompting someone to complain about innovation clutter. But mostly they compete with the past and almost always win.

Love sees most clearly in the aftermath of loss, betrayal and pain, when the cynical smirk seems most appropriate. Love does not always see how to restore that which is broken, but it always has eyes for how life can find a way. Love in the aftermath of loss is tuned with the sensitivity of a bruise.

I tend to hang around with groups of people with hopes verging on grandiosity. On many days we actually do think about world peace, saving the planet, and about the least of these. This is good; what else should grownups think about? The challenge is that we are deceived into thinking that the hero of the story always tends to be...us...because we can see the possibilities and those possibilities tend to be extrapolated from our kinds of skills. We can see the future and it looks like more of us at an even larger scale: Health insurance for all (so that everybody could come to our great hospitals!), public health unleashed to prevent everything possible to prevent, education so widespread and enlightened that nobody would ever do anything dumb again.

History exaggerates what has happened and undervalues what could have happened just as easily. And it says little about what is possible, what has not yet happened. Emmanuel Kant insisted that the possibilities are just as real as the actualities (McGaughey & Cochrane, 2017). The possibilities are all we can do anything about. The point is to give our life to the possibilities that allow life to emerge with the most mercy and justice possible. History also exaggerates the power of boundaries and differences, projecting today's identities inappropriately backward across time, giving them far more power than they deserve. The actual testimony of life is all about dissolving boundaries, especially the ones in our head.

Some of the boundaries in our heads are extremely helpful and protective. The weak, very young, minorities, and the easily violated live on the strength of the perimeter that defines their life space. The point is that that perimeter is not really there in any physical sense. This is why it has to be consciously defined and ritually enforced. This can be either immoral or noble; it depends on who is being protected from whom or what. Professional standards for clergy, counselors, and caregivers protect the easily violated. Apartheid and race laws protected those with privileges that defied the social gravity and the naturally generative buoyancy of diversity.

Generative people see difference, head that direction, and cross right over. They tend to do so because they have learned they'll probably like what and who is on the other side of whatever boundary others say divides. It is important not to exaggerate the nobility involved. It's more about curiosity and playfulness. I don't think that humanity spread across the globe because of drab duty. Far more likely the generative ones in the tribe just went over the next mountain, down the river, and around the bend because, well, just because that's what they do.

Generative people tend to live across whatever divides. They don't just think, read, or talk across the lines; they live in relationships that cross lines. You have probably taken, at some point (usually a low one), one of the ever-growing menu of personality analyses. I'm the type who can't remember my type, whether it be DISC (Dominance, Inducement, Submission, Compliance), Myers-Briggs, Enneagram, or the dozen others I've taken along the way. I think that one's persona is more like the biome in the gut with accumulated complexity that is nearly infinitely nuanced, mostly hidden beneath the four, nine, five, or dozen letters. So don't look for a type. I'm not a physician, psychologist, social worker, nutritionist, therapist, or counselor of any sort. Not a fitness trainer, sports coach, financial analyst, or leadership guru. I am the very last one who will ever give you a list of recommended behaviors. But I notice patterns in those living generative lives that may resonate with what you've seen in generative lives around you. It may remind you of yourself, the bones growing under the vines others mistake for you.

Letting the Light In

History also exaggerates the dangers and damages of failure. The breaks and discontinuities turn on the lights of caution and trust, humility and possibility. It is possible to keep track of an ever-growing list of mistakes, determining not to make them again, and miss the ever-beginning story. TC and I have both been married to other hugely decent people we still hold in high regard, a classically sprawling modern family. To avoid some of the first-family politics, we decided to get married in Cape Town amid a crazy assortment of friends gathered in a kind of a treehouse high above a long beach pointing toward the Cape called Hope. We had asked Sepetla Molapo, a bright and mystical academic now at University of Pretoria, who worked as a graduate researcher on the early ARHAP teams, to bring some words to augment the sacramental efforts of our friend and Methodist pastor, Mark Stephenson. Sepetla is African, which is to say that he takes words and stories seriously. He told of the expectations he was raised with in a noble Lethoso family—that he would marry and carry forward the lineage. He didn't find anyone to marry after high school, so went straight on to college. Still no one appeared, so graduate school was the next step instead of children. Another degree and the realization that perhaps family would never happen for him. "And then, I received an email from

Gary and TC and I realized that anything can happen! Anything at all!" The transitions in life are where we see what is possible with ever-new clarity—what can be healed and with what we must reconcile by living.

Medicine as Reconciliation

The word "medicine" goes back to Egypt, finding its roots in the idea of mediation and reconciliation. Healing is bridging over, restoring vital relationship. At a molecular level, this is the purpose of herbs and now pharmaceuticals. Pills do not and cannot give life where there is none. Healing works with—mediates—living human life to find its way, the tendon back to the bone, the virus back to balance. The work of mediating—reconciling—is as complex as the living phenomenon.

We may wish to hand the work of this kind of mediation to others. Dr. Robin Womeodu, the Chief Medical Officer of Methodist Le Bonheur Healthcare, tells of people, convinced of the magical properties of medicine, dropping their momma off at the hospital every winter to get her fixed back up. Some physicians like that kind of expectation—the elevation and distance it brings. But it deprives all involved—mom, kids, and doctor—of healing. Some public health officers like the idea that they could fix a whole community—if only they had the money. Healing at a large scale is mediating and reconciling the life of the whole living thing with its own connections, coherence, agency, generativity, and hope.

Reconciliation is not a trick that you do to somebody else; it sees the boundaries and knows them to be a lie. We start from our side of the barrier, recognizing our own fraught, but hopeful, humanity. That first move—toward our own transitions—teaches us humility so that we can see the possibilities in others' complex lives. Health is not something you do to somebody else; neither is justice, nor education, nor recovery from addiction, nor recovery from crime. These are all the names of relationships that can be open to generative possibilities beyond the cold facts of steel, electrons, and the past. Life finds a way, but rarely—very, very rarely—one life at a time. It finds a way across lives that find ways into relationships that are reconciled and generative.

After Larry Pray's stroke, he found his way through that journey and wrote an extraordinary book, Thresholds (2012), with his neurologist David Gumm, about "connecting body and soul after brain injury." He describes a young maple that caught his eye:

Its branches were almost jet black, and its leaves ablaze in Indian Yellow, whose brilliant light echoed between them. All of a sudden, several of the leaves let go. There was no particular reason, no wind, no passing car, no kids shaking the branches. They just let go and began fluttering to the ground. In a moment or two, hundreds of leaves joined the three or four that first fell. And almost before the newcomers touched the ground, virtually every leaf on the entire tree surrendered to the touch of fall. In a minute or two, the tree was bare and the ground was a pool of yellow leaves (p. 19).

Larry understood his stroke to be like that, but I think it may be one way to think of our lives, which are given a season and find beauty from one cycle to the next, living right up to the very edge.

History deceives us about the power of the anxieties and differences that divide us. The cracks visible in each others' lives let in the light of humanity where we can see commonality in real ways. The transitions give us a chance to be human and recognize another human by simply honoring and speaking to the reality of a life transition. Imagine someone with whom you radically disagree; after their marriage or divorce or remarriage, imagine making a simple phone call or writing a note (not email and, God save us, not text!) saying you noticed and wanted them to know. You have to go beyond a stupid one-dimensional health lens; it doesn't help much to think of the transition as purely biological or physical. Nobody in Lesotho would do that, and even an American can see that a twisted ankle has psychological, social, and spiritual implications—just ask any aging tennis player. On this occasion, do not think of health as an opportunity to see how you can fix something but as one of the zillion opportunities to observe the cracks and bends where the common humanity shines through. A daughter with a broken arm, a sister celebrating a year of recovery, a neighbor rejoicing in a clean remission report, a nephew with a reoccurrence, a colleague losing 20 pounds, another walking after knee replacement. Being lost; being found. Common. Human.

These are things that happen in life and can be brought into focus by seeing them through the lenses of life—connections, coherence, agency, generativity, and hope. A crisis in another life is not the time for theory, but theory can help you see the pathos and possibility clearly enough to find your voice or a touch of common humanity. A transitional crisis is not the time for therapy or instruction, much less blame. It is a time to see clearly the common frailty in our lives and speak to the commonality we share.

A community has transitions, too, that offer up opportunities for humanity, if seen through the eyes of realistic love: the abandoned quarry turned into a park, the drop in infant morality rates after decades of struggle, the outpouring of volunteers after the flood. The negative cracks, if addressed in the kind of love that does not rejoice in evil, can be spoken, too. The flood of addictions as it shifts from prescriptions to imported heroin shatters families, neighborhoods, and crashes entire community systems. Spoken in love, the crisis crosses boundaries. Other crises seem harder for love to enter because of the attribution of blame: carbon-based climate change being one obvious example. Many of the polarizing arguments are socially constructed and reinforced by those who benefit from the divide. Tell the truth, but in ways that allow the light of common humanity to shine in.

Commonality of the Broken

Generative lives sprawl into and across every possible human definition of separateness. We are attracted to and thrive on the life that emerges constantly on the edges where difference touches, where life grows, changes, and adapts to what is possible.

Of course, the actuality of our broken human reality is that we are driven by differences of language, class, education, and all sorts of leftover identities. Each of us is raised amid our own detritus of whatever cultural stuff and clutter meant "home." I was raised in a politely racist Methodist family, and I remember hearing things that would make me reel today. Every South African white person has stories almost impossible to share. Most of my friends of color have images like poison inside them, too. Rev. Richard Joyner, of Conetoe, North Carolina, tells of working for decades to get the "less than" self-images out of his head. He told a local hospital he could not accept their grant because it was dangerous to be in a "less than" relationship. He'd do a contract to sell food raised on his farm, but not accept a grant.

Philosopher Immanuel Kant knew that this actuality is real, just not complete. The possibilities are just as real as the actualities, and we see their sprouts emerging in places you'd never expect (which is where you should always expect them). Italian Protestant Christians wade into the waters off Sicily, risking their physical and political lives to save illegal Muslim Africans. They make the possibility of justice become just as real as the cold water and the cold-hearted authorities. The Waldensians helping immigrants now were hunted by Catholic priests and government powers for centuries, only receiving the legal rights of full Italian citizenship in the 1980s, along with the Jews. Their progeny know about the deadly wickedness of separation and have always found possibilities across the actualities others protect. They lived in actual oppression and cruelty for nine centuries. The possibilities of mercy and justice were strong enough to hold fast until the time came when their love could bear fruit in justice for others.

Living that way generates life's own possibilities. But it may take more than a handful of lifetimes. The Pope finally came to the home church of the Waldensians in 2015 to apologize for the centuries of persecution. It was about time, but everyone was still pleasantly surprised it happened when it did. In Sicily, local politicians still easily exploit racial and religious fears to make the Waldensians' poeisis illegal. They feast like raptors on what looks like naïve vulnerability. Who knows if their feast is only for a season, an election cycle or two, or maybe four or six. The Waldensians have seen it before. They have learned over the centuries to trust in the generative power of possible relationships lived into with hope and confidence. Life is what works. It is the only thing that works for the human journey.

Life is stronger and smarter than all that would contain and defeat it, precisely because of its quality of loveliness. The very weakest and most vulnerable of all human capacities—loveliness—is precisely what works to always find a way. Every master of torture and shame thinks their capacity to hurt those we love is our weakness. In the moment of radical intimacy, when it is one master and one wife or daughter or grandson under threat, they are always right. All the gorgeous mountains and material wonders in the world are not worth the suffering of those we love. But the radical proves the general. What would we not give away to protect the hopes of the whole lovely world? What would we not give up in order to protect the whole?

In the end of our individual days, we find that the aggressive military metaphors are deceivers. It's not about war, but about life finding a way as it always does. Chaos does fight back, but its only real tactic is to make us forget our creative imagination. How do we avoid fighting back against that kind of fighting back?

There is no stronger imagination that that powered by love. It can make us see possibilities that are beyond available evidence—that turn out to be real. What does it mean to love in the context of the snarly and conflicted world of human systems—not romance but committees? The best description of committee-quality love comes from one of the least romantic writers of all time, Paul. The irony is that his paean to love in his letter to the Corinthians has been used in a large percentage of all Christian weddings for centuries. He didn't even like marriage, considering it a distracting nuisance only for those without the will and focus to give their lives entirely to work. But he found himself exasperated by an impossibly grumpy and conflicted church in the rough seaport town of Corinth. What social movement could have less going for it than that early gaggle of mostly women, slaves, and outcasts making up the early churches? Paul, who knew weakness as only a former bully ever can, spoke into these fragile networks offering up love.

I think he'd approve of my adaptation of his words, partly because it is unlikely to be used in many weddings.

> To Whom It May Concern:
>
> From: Life
>
> If I speak in the voice of powerful people or spirits but do not have loving kindness, I am only a distracting noise. If I have predictive data and interdisciplinary analytics that give me confidence to move mountains of poverty, but am not kind, I am nothing. If I proudly commit to radical levels of community benefit and take on huge obligations for the health of the public, but am not humbled by love, I do nothing.
>
> The love that life needs is patient and kind. It does not envy, it does not boast, it is not proud. It does not

dishonor others, it is not self-seeking, it is not easily angered, it keeps no record of wrongs. Loving kindness does not delight in evil but rejoices with the truth. It always protects, always trusts, always hopes, always perseveres.

Love never gives up. Where we have predictions and projections, they will cease; where there are speeches, they will be forgotten; where there is knowledge, it will be eclipsed by other knowledge. For we know in part and we predict in part, but when living complexity comes, what is partial disappears. When we were young in our work we talked like beginners, and reasoned like beginners. When we became a grownups, we put the ways of childhood behind. For now we see only a dimly as if looking through a smoky haze; then we shall see it all directly. Now we know a bit; then we may know fully, even as our own lives will be fully known.

And now these three remain in life: faith, hope and love. But above and beyond and after all is love.

This kind of gritty love draws our curiosity toward the future, to what has not yet happened. It is hard to see with an imagination tethered like vines to the past. We give too much authority to what has already happened and too little to what still might.

I shared this adapted version of Paul's counsel with the leadership of the advocacy group of the American Public Health Association. These are folks who stare into the loud mouth of chaos every day. One asked, with no small edge, "Reverend Gunderson...(long pause)...do you love tobacco companies?" These are the agents of more death every single year than the death camps managed in all of World War II. We live less than 400 yards from where the very first cigarette machine was made, which propelled an oddly cumbersome smoking process into the efficiently addictive deadly process it is today. This is how chaos fights, by deceiving us into wanting things that destroy our bodies, that drag enormous medical debt into the lives of our families, that waste money, land, time, and energy for nothing at all. Love hates such deception but does not mirror its methods in order to resist. Love gives us the power to find common purpose and the courage to speak the truth. Most important of all, it gives us a way to avoid being sucked into the undertow of chaos.

Chaos often wins—decade after deadly decade—but it is not delusional to observe that it always eventually undermines itself and ultimately fails. Stephen Pinker (2011) has meticulously documented the reality that over time human beings have trended toward less and less organized violence and more and more tolerance. This offers no big comfort to a neighborhood ripped apart by gangs and corrupt government officers. But it is a comfort to those trusting in the power of life to find a way.

In any given place where life is breaking through and chaos is fighting back, it will be the weakest and most vulnerable—whatever that means in a particular place and time—who will suffer. It takes discernment to recognize who is weak in your particular context. It might be the honest city council person or the compassionate jailer or perhaps the pediatrician who just can't look away. They might not be vulnerable in the way you expect, so you'll need to look closely in order to be useful.

Love is the greatest virtue because it is the name of a relationship that defeats our blinding individualism and just-as-blinding objectivity. Love sees the unpredictable consequences of life more accurately than history because it knows that the future is not determined yet. The most important thing about the future is that it comes out of the utterly unpredictable expression of collective creative imagination. Nothing ignites the imagination like love.

STEP 8

Risk Life

There, I think you've got it. That's what my mother told me one day. At the time, I thought she was dying and asked her for some last bit of wisdom just for me. Nope. She said she'd already told me everything and was pretty sure I'd remember it when I needed to. I'm pretty sure you've got most everything you might need, too. You've learned:

- To speak the language of life
- To look beyond imagined boundaries
- How life works
- How you can work with life
- What matters most
- How to fight chaos

All of this will work. So go ahead and risk your life.

You will find that life will hold you aloft if you trust it—just as a young hawk learns to trust the wind. The nest is safer but wings are for the wind high above the ridge. Humans do not soar on wings. We step here and then there, sometimes backing up to go forward.

While the hawk rises on the currents, we find our way amid committees, memos, and long tangled conversations, filled with all the ambiguities of words, silences, and glances. And we don't have eyes like a hawk, either, which can see a mouse flinch from hundreds of feet above. We miss even the most obvious things, especially about ourselves. So we must help each other.

Human life is not impressive as experiments go. We are hardly a blip amid the tectonic wanderings of the continents. The cold-blooded raptors had hundreds of millions of years compared to our handful. Our brief thousands are an imperceptible layer of archeological dust. You'd have to admit we're not having our best century either. The days are late and the time closing. But maybe it's not too late, if we give our lives over to life. See if the wind of the Spirit doesn't remind you of what your hands, voice, and mind are for. I'm asking you to risk life. But it's not really a risk to do what you are made to do.

The beauty of the natural world touches me deeply, not because it is perfect, but because it is perfectly adapted and still adapting to dynamic processes. Fred Smith asked me a profound question as I raved about the beauty of the lions I had seen in the wild in Africa, so very different from those seen in a zoo. They were perfectly adapted to the tall winter grass that shifted in the breeze, the same tawny brown as their manes. Their eyes were ever tuned so as never to miss a thing, and their practiced social web was so subtle and strategic. Fred quietly asked, "What are we perfectly adapted for?" Good question. My answer? Life.

Live it out. Give it all away—every bit —and you will be an agent of life. This choice does not make you tame, tepid, or patient. It may get you killed. But it might also open and hold open some social space that gives life a chance.

Some reading this book might find the word "God" something to trip over. If you want to align yourself with the creative spirit of life (known by the Jewish people as YHWH, but perhaps otherwise by you), then love mercy, do justice, and walk humbly before that greater, wider, deeper, ever-flowing phenomenon that is carrying you. It's not yours; indeed, you can't even imagine the edges of it. So walk in grateful awe. Do that. Otherwise, your humble-walking will be merely role-playing—one more cleverness amid a clutter of clever life tricks designed to accomplish something. Life shifts our attention to the ground on which we stand, that we did not make; to the air that holds the hawk, that the hawk did not make. Walk humbly before the mysteries you are meant to serve, not as if they are something that you created.

This kind of humility makes us fierce and bold, and allows us to sit down like Rosa Parks did, to wait like Nelson Mandela did for 26 years, and to walk like John Lewis did down the slope of the Edmund Pettus Bridge in Selma, Alabama, with eyes wide open to what could—and would—come next. And to what is still possible in the great beyond.

Go to the Limit of Your Risk

There is no way to know exactly what bridge calls you. Whatever it is, find it and cross it. In the world of health, we speak of people operating at the "top of their license"—stretching to the appropriate limit of their training and experience, and then knowing where the rest of the team needs to pick up. In poeisis, we must each go to the limit of our own risk, stretching beyond safety to open and hold open space for others. That means that people who have more should risk more. Those with privilege, resources, reputation, health, mobility, networks, gifts of language, or time should risk more. These things are not yours, anyway. Don't be too proud; you are not the living seed. You are just good loam and the seed needs that to have a chance.

I wish I could tell you that the way I've sketched for you will give you a long journey through the pleasures of the world. It might. But life doesn't work that way every time in every individual life. Others sat, waited, and walked long before Rosa, Nelson, and John, whose names we know and honor. Each of those who went before had lives filled with pain and loss. This is the humble knowledge we actually have—not the false cleverness of some canny trick that gets us stuff. The only sure thing is that if you give your life away to something greater than your clutter of stuff, life will take your gift and invest it in others.

Lend Yourself Gracefully

Foresters continue to debate about whether fire is good or bad. It's bad for this particular tree, of course, so we short-lived humans try to put out fires whenever we can. But the thing called a "forest" is a phenomenon measured over hundreds of years. This is so long that a particular bird—the Black-backed Woodpecker—was perfectly adapted to the charred trees left after a fire. Some of our greatest hopes are like burned-over forests. Some of us have ideas or a dream adapted perfectly to a big, burned-over wasteland—I'm thinking of the square miles of Detroit, Memphis, or St. Louis. The human journey is not so fragile as to depend on an unbroken string of success. It often cycles through times of great suffering and terrific loss. Maybe like forests, we need the fire. I don't know. But I know we are built to survive fire. The United Nations, born in the Muir Woods, channeled a hope fired in the horrors of a global war. I expect that the current angry mess in which chaos is having its way with us, will call out some new dream, too.

Henry David Thoreau's last public lecture, "Autumnal Tints," explains how trees—in particular leaves—teach us how to lend ourselves gracefully to that which lives beyond us. Richard Higgins (2017) recounts Thoreau's words in Thoreau and the Language of Trees:

"They that soared so loftily, how contentedly they return to dust again, and are laid low, resigned to lie and decay at the foot of the tree, and afford nourishment to new generations" (p. 93).

As I write this, Larry Pray is still improbably writing poetry with the handful of synapses he's got left to work with. He is hanging on more like one of the tenacious beech leaves that cling long into winter than one of the maples he loved. He will live right up until he won't—and then he will continue to nurture those of us remaining as his life resonates in ours.

Isn't that what any grownup hopes to do?

You measure a life by what it generates, not by what it grasps. At the end you release the grasp anyway as all the physical stuff cycles away. But what you generate remains alive, the tough reality of faith, hope, and love. You don't know how many generative years you might have. The point is not to try to save them up but to pour them out. Jesus turned out to have 33. I'm not sure how to do the arithmetic for the years since his last fish dinner by the lake, a few days after the cross and stone-rolling. He's a special case, anyway, but worth noticing for His almost casually generous style and laser vision allowing him to notice those in society who were "the least." He lived it out and gave it all away.

Dr. King had a half dozen more years, never even making it to the age of 40. He was less perfect than Jesus and did not rise again from the grave. He has now been dead for longer than he lived, but who could doubt that he continues to nurture confidence in the long arc of history? Gandhi generated life for 78 years, his last couple dozen marked with more humility than the earlier ones as he lived to see his young hopes find root in the tangled soil of a new government. He did not die in his sleep, but he certainly lived in his hopes. Rosa Parks lived to 92, long enough to see a black mayor and police chief in Birmingham but not quite long enough to see the first black president just over the horizon.

You probably will not be the CEO of a big thing, although that could happen; stranger things do. More likely is that you'll be a planner for a small mountain county with a dumpy office. Or you may be a professor in a religion department in some college without a big name. You might feel ignored while the administration thunders off after donors for their snazzy new business school. Maybe you'll be a pediatrician hoping to draw kids into one community scheme after another. Maybe you're a pastor or a priest—or married to one—and you will only ever be known in the intimate spaces of a small town. Maybe you're an economist drawn beyond your discipline into the service of hope that makes all your colleagues think you odd. Maybe you've been an obvious star from youth with a crackling intelligence that drew support from every kind of scholarship and research grant along the way until you found yourself succeeding in the very machine your spirit didn't want. Maybe you're 17 years old, with clear eyes and a full heart, and you don't want to wait to give your life to a world that needs people on the risky edges of hope now. Hope now that you'll be known by the hopes for which you risked your life.

Jesus found Himself in wild places. He found something more preposterous than all the canyons on earth: that amid all the harshness, fragility, and loss, loving kindness survives. Humans care and care for each other, even as blood, race, wealth, politics, religion, and ethnicity fall like nameless stone from the cliffs. The rocks fall; the kindness survives. What could be more obvious than the fact that everyone who lived in the past also died, felt pain, and knew sorrow? We know it for ourselves and we know it for all those we love, too. Bitter resignation makes sense. But generation after generation, we find loving kindness. Life is fragile, short, and harsh; therefore, do not cease to be radical in your love of the world God so loves.

Going Higher...Backwards

In 1963, a tall and skinny high school sophomore could not high jump within a foot of his own height. He failed to qualify even for school competitions, which required a starting jump of at least five feet. Like everyone since the Greeks more than a thousand years ago, he was taught to approach the bar at a run, pushing off with one foot and diving over it like a cruise missile. Today, he would probably just take up video gaming, but this was Portland, Oregon, in the early sixties so he had little choice but to find another way up and over the bar. "I knew I had to change my body position and that's what started first the revolution, and over the next two years, the evolution," he recounts. First he tried running toward the bar at an angle, then approaching sideways, then—improbably—he found a way to push off while twisting backward and using his legs to flop himself over to the other side of the bar. It looked ridiculous. And it worked. He set his school record the next year and the state record the year after. A not insignificant part of the story is that this young man's highflying backwardness coincided with a movement to change the material in the landing pit from wood chips to thick foam rubber. Without this softer landing he would have certainly suffered brain damage at some point as he landed on his head from seven feet in the air.

In 1968, Dick Fosbury won the Olympic gold medal in Mexico City, with British announcers chuckling the whole time. Right up until he cleared the bar at seven feet three and a quarter inches he was regarded with disdain; one article branded him the "laziest high jumper in the world." A few stubborn old timers stuck to the old "straddle" method for some years, but it quickly fell out of fashion in favor of the much more efficient and successful Fosbury Flop. Anyone straddling the high jump bar today would be regarded as a hopeless fossil. Even the British would laugh.

It turns out that humans are built to jump over high objects... backwards.

Today we face a very high bar indeed. We are not playing a game for a little metal medallion but for the survival of our melting planet in the name of everyone you love as well as everyone whose names you'll never hear. Anyone who is not daunted by this task understands neither data nor our perilous consumptive momentum. A little bit better and a little quicker will not be enough. We need a whole different pace, height, and method if we are to clear this bar.

We need to turn around.

I'm not confident that we have much cushioning to work with, given the thinning ice, rising water, and animals on the run everywhere. But our relative wealth, even if most of it is concentrated in relatively uncaring hands, gives us something to work with. We may be able to find our footing in a new way that enables us to turn around and start moving toward life. We may have just enough time—if we don't skip over the "figuring it out" part. Fosbury, now an engineer, was thoughtful, not casual, in his figuring. He developed a whole new way of talking so that he could experiment with a whole new way of moving.

But first he had to stop thinking about the old way. We do, too. Wayne Merritt, who taught me Greek, said that Jesus' message was that you will know the truth and the truth will make you odd.

Let's go higher...backwards. Let's do the counterintuitive thing that no one expects. Let's speak life.

Truth Will Make You Odd

Jesus came out of the wilderness and gave Himself to healing—and never stopped, not even for the Sabbath. He said that He would stop healing when His Parent did. How preposterous, how human, how holy. We don't know whether to laugh at Him or cry for how strange that sounds to us. And what did He do besides healing pretty much everyone who found Him? What does He tell His movement to do? He doesn't provide a box of tricks. He gives a way to live, and what a crazy way: How happy are the humble, those who know sorrow, who claim nothing, who are starving for goodness. Here He gets specific: How happy are the merciful (not merely desiring to show mercy but doing it); and so too those who are sincere and those who do the work of peacemaking. And, here He gets even worse: Happy are those who suffer persecution for the cause of goodness, especially when people tweet about them and make things up entirely. If you suffer for living a true life of radical generosity, how lucky you are!

This, Jesus says, is what salt is for, what light is for, what life is for.

He keeps the radical pedal down, which must have been disconcerting to those just looking for some free medical care. Jesus said that anger is as bad as murder! Anyone who calls someone a fool commits a serious crime, and anyone who says someone is lost is himself heading straight to the fire. I happen to call a particular partisan group lost fools, which makes me guilty of both of those transgressions. I wish Jesus would be more reasonable and supportive of my movement. But He never gets more reasonable; He only gets worse. "Don't tell people that God will guarantee your promise, no eye for an eye, no hitting back, and if the cops make you do one mile, give them another. And give to anybody who asks anything."

On and on, page after page, without a single tip about how to beat Herod, his palace "glamourotti," and his ever-grinning children. "Jesus...is...impossible," every king and king-hater alike has said for two millennia.

The prophet Isaiah wrote, "Comfort My people, for in the darkness we have a seen a great light" (Isaiah 9:2). But the light of Jesus is not the light we want. It is not a way out or a way over, but a way through; a way to live day by day, year by year, even generation after generation after generation, if we have to, waiting for the promises of God for mercy and justice to be realized. And what do we do while we wait for the big show? Go do mercy and some justice, that's what. Jesus' promise is that you and I can live this way, The Way, the only way that gives life a chance at all.

Come and be part of the end of all fear, especially the fear of all death and the power to kill. Come and give your body and mind to The Way that leads to life. Give yourself away, every bit, and you will feel the life flow where once you held tight to your little fears and hopes. Give it away, every bit. Be part of the healing and don't start big. Before you make a big holy show of it, think of your brother, sister, former spouse, or left-behind friend; go make peace with them first. Come away from the anger and scheming. Quit bargaining and holding your minor gains as if they will last. Live this way now and you will find life flowing freely, abundant, overflowing beyond all measure at all.

You might say that it didn't work out so well for Jesus or for those who bet their lives on His words. Herod won without a recount. Pilot, two clicks meaner, won too. Most kings do most of the time. But take a look at the end of the Jesus story. The story of the boats and fishers is so good that it shows up in all four gospels in four different ways. In the tender days after the assassination and the scattering of the disciples, the fishermen went back to fishing for fish. Simon Peter, Thomas, Nathanael, Zebedee's sons, and two other disciples were hiding at the lake north of Mt. Airy. Peter announced that he was going fishing and, since nobody wanted to be left behind, they all tumbled into the boat. They stayed out all night and caught nothing. They headed back in the next morning, even more discouraged than when they had started. Worse, they were also hungry.

Jesus watched from the beach across the early mist and called, "Children, have you caught anything to eat?" (No, of course not.) "Cast on the right side where it's deeper and you'll find some." They netted so many they couldn't haul them in. John reports 153 fish, which is like counting the beer bottles left on the lawn after any other football team in the southeast beats Carolina. Peter sure didn't bother counting the fish. Naked, he jumped out of the boat and pushed his way a hundred yards through waist-deep water to get to his beloved friend.

Listen to the tenderness of the One who calls us into a preposterous Way of generous vulnerability. This is a Savior who knows we need to eat as much as we need hope—and that we need hope as much as we need breakfast.

The generative One does not give us a way to beat the mean and violent, but neither does He counsel us to give way to liars and schemers. He gives us The Way to be different from them. They have no power to stop you from living The Way of Life. Their castles are as froth on the waves. You are drawing from a deeper place, carried by a deeper current, stronger even than one that can cut through stone like the Colorado River. The healer is here among us as we fish, and type, and give away our lives in healing, or teaching, or raising hope through art or kindness. Give yourself to life-giving now, not later. Hold back nothing for a safer or smarter time. Life is at hand, says the generative One. I think He meant that life is at your very fingertips.

Jesus had started a charcoal fire on the beach, expecting the haul, toasting some bread to go along with it. "Bring me some of the fish; y'all need some breakfast."

Savor that. And then give it away.

Endnotes

Here We Go

Faulkner, W. (1951). *Requiem for a Nun*. New York: Random House.

Gunderson, G. R., with Pray, L. (2009). *Leading Causes of Life: Five Fundamentals to Change the Way You Live Your Life*. Nashville: Abingdon Press.

Step 1

Capon, R.F. (1996). *The Astonished Heart: Reclaiming the Good News from the Lost-and-Found of Church History*. Grand Rapids, MI/Cambridge, U.K.: Wm. B. Eerdmans Publishing Company.

Cutts, T.F., & Cochrane, J.R. (Eds). (2016). *Stakeholder Health: Insights from New Systems of Health*. USA: FaithHealth Innovations, Inc.

Hale, Lori Brandt. (2018). "Is this a Bonhoeffer Moment?" *Sojourners*, February 2018.

Step 2

Church-Health System Partnership Facilitates Transitions from Hospital to Home for Urban, Low-Income African Americans, Reducing Mortality, Utilization, and Costs. Retrieved from https://innovations. ahrq.gov/profiles/church- health-system-partnership-facilitates-transitions-hospital-home-urban-low-income.

Barnes, P.B., Cutts, T.F., Dickinson, S.B., Guo, H., Squires, D., Bowman, S., & Gunderson, G. (2014). "Methods for Managing and Analyzing Electronic Medical Records: A Formative Examination of a Hospital-Congregation Based Intervention." *Population Health Management,*

October 17(5): 279-286.

Barry, J. M. (1998). *Rising Tide: The Great Mississippi Flood of 1927 and How it Changed America*. New York: Simon & Schuster.

Bauman, Z. (2000). *Liquid Modernity*. Cambridge: Polity Press.

Bohm, D. (2002). *Wholeness and the Implicate Order*. London; New York: Routledge.

Germond, P., & Cochrane, J.R. (2010). "Healthworlds: Conceptualizing Landscapes of Health and Healing." *Sociology*, 44:307-324.

Gleick, James. (1988). *Chaos: Making a New Science*. New York: Penguin Books.

Gunderson, G. R., & Pray, L. (2004). *Boundary Leaders: Leadership Skills for People of Faith*. Minneapolis: Fortress Press.

Kreuter, M.W., De Rosa C., Howze, E.H., Baldwin, G.T. (2004). "Understanding Wicked Problems: A Key to Advancing Environmental Health Promotion." *Health Education & Behavior*, Aug. 31(4):441-54.

Moin, P., & Kim, J. (1997). "Tackling Turbulence with Supercomputers." *Scientific American*, 276(1): 62-69. Retrieved May 2010, from http://turb.seas.ucla.edu/~jkim/ sciam/turbulence.html.

Salk, Jonas. (1973). *The Survival of the Wisest*. New York: Harper & Row.

Step 3
Antonovsky, A. (1987). *Unraveling the Mystery of Health: How People Manage Stress and Stay Well*. San Francisco: Jossey-Bass.

Benn, C. (2014). "Faith, Health, and Peace: Seeking the Basic Right to Good Health for All God's Children." Keynote address at the Lake

Junaluska Peace Conference. Lake Junaluska, NC, March 27, 2014.

Dickinson, E. (1862). "Hope is the Thing with Feathers." https://www. poets.org/poetsorg/poem/hope-thing-feathers-254. Retrieved March 13, 2018.

McKibben, B. (2011). *Eaarth: Making a Life on a Tough New Planet.* New York: Henry Holt and Company.

King, M.L. (1963). Speech given at Western Michigan University on Dec. 18, 1963. http://wmich.edu/sites/default/files/attachments/ MLK.pdf. Retrieved on March 13, 2018.

Salk, Jonas. (1973). *The Survival of the Wisest.* New York: Harper & Row.

Wilkinson, R., & Pickett, K. (2009). *The Spirit Level: Why Greater Equality Makes Societies Stronger.* New York: Bloomsbury Press.

Young, N. (1970). "Don't Let it Bring You Down." https://en.wikipedia. org/wiki/Don%27t_Let_It_Bring_You_Down. Retrieved March 13, 2018.

Step 4
Alinksy, S. http://www.azquotes.com/author/247-Saul_Alinsky?p=3. Retrieved March 7, 2018.

Cohen, L. (1992). "Anthem." https://www.bing.com/search?q=leona rd+cohen+song+anthem&src=IE-SearchBox&FORM=IESR3A. Retrieved March 12, 2018.

Cooperrider, D.L., & Srivastva, S. (1987). "Appreciative Inquiry in Organizational Life." In Woodman, R. W., & Pasmore, W.A. (Eds.) *Research In Organizational Change and Development*, Vol. 1: 129 169. Stamford, CT: JAI Press.

Crosby, M. C. (2006). *The American Plague: The Untold Story of Yellow Fever, the Epidemic that Shaped Our History.* New York: Berkley Books.

Cutts, T., Langdon, S., Meza, F. R., Hochwalt, B., Pichardo-Geisinger, R., Sowell, B, et al. (2016). Community Health Asset Mapping Partnership Engages Hispanic/Latino Health Seekers and Providers. *North Carolina Medical Journal,* 77(3), 160-167. doi:10.18043/ncm.77.3.160.

Gunderson, G. R. (1997). *Deeply Woven Roots: Improving the Quality of Life in Your Community.* Minneapolis: Augsburg Fortress Press.

Gunderson, G. R., with Pray, L. (2009). *Leading Causes of Life: Five Fundamentals to Change the Way You Live Your Life.* Nashville: Abingdon Press.

Interfaith Health Program. (1993). *Faith & Health.* Atlanta: Carter Center.

Kania, J., & Kramer, M. (2011). "Collective Impact." *Stanford Social Innovation Review,* Winter. http://ssir.org/articles/entry/collective_impact.

Kretzmann, J.P., & McKnight, J.L. (1993). *Building Communities from the Inside Out: A Path Toward Finding and Mobilizing a Community's Assets.* Evanston, IL: Institute for Policy Research, pp. 1-11.

Munnecke, T. "On Toasters and Cats." https://wiki.p2pfoundation.net/Tom_Munnecke. Retrieved on March 12, 2018.

Murthy, V. (2015). "Remarks from the U.S. Surgeon General." Presented at Partners in Health: Aligning Clinical Systems, Faith and Community Assets. April 15-16, 2015. Washington, D.C.: The White House.

Salk, Jonas. (1973). *The Survival of the Wisest.* New York: Harper & Row.

Wesley, J. (1761). *Primitive Physick Or an Easy and Natural Method of Curing Most Diseases*. University of Lausanne: W. Strahan.

Wolff, T, Minkler, M., Wolfe., S.M., et al. (2016). "Collaborating for Equity and Justice: Moving Beyond Collective Impact." *Nonprofit Quarterly*, Winter 2016. 42-53.

Wolford, B. (2014). "Murmuration: How Starlings Dance Across the Sky in Perfect Unison." *International Science Times*, January 23, 2014. http://www.isciencetimes.com/articles/6725/20140123/murmuration-starlings-dance-sky-perfect-unison.htm. Retrieved on March 12, 2018.

Wright, F.L. (1908). "In the Cause of Architecture." http://www.learn.columbia.edu/courses/arch20/pdf/art_hum_reading_51.pdf. Retrieved on March 12, 2018.

Step 5
Beyerhaus, P. (1987). *The Kairos Document: Challenge or Danger to the Church? A Critical Theological Assessment of South African People's Theology*. South Africa: Gospel Defence League.

Cochrane, J.R., Schmid, B., Cutts, T. (Eds.). (2011). *When Religion and Health Align: Mobilising Religious Health Assets for Transformation*. Dorpspruit, South Africa: Cluster Publications.

Gillespie, M. A. (1984). *Hegel, Heidegger, and the Ground of History*. Chicago: University of Chicago Press.

Holman, S. (2015). *Beholden: Religion, Global Health, and Human Rights*. New York: Oxford University Press.

Step 6
Begos, K., Deaver, D., Railey, J., Sexton, S., & Lombardo, P. (2012). *Against Their Will: North Carolina's Sterilization Program and the Campaign for Reparations*. Apalachicola, FL: Gray Oak Books.

Campbell, J. (1991). In Osbon, D. (Ed.), *Reflections on the Art of Living: A Joseph Campbell Companion*. New York: HarperCollins Publishers.

Cutts, T., & Gunderson, G. (2017). "The North Carolina Way: Emerging Healthcare System and Faith Community Partnerships." *Development in Practice,* Vol. 27(5): 719-732.

Fricchione, G. L. (2002). "Separation, Attachment, and Altruistic Love: The Evolutionary Basis for Medical Caring." In S. G. Post, L. G.

Underwood, J. P Schloss, & W. B. Hurlbut (Eds.) *Altruism and Altruistic Love: Science, Philosophy, and Religion in Dialogue,* (pp. 346-361). New York: Oxford University Press.

Gunderson, G., Cutts, T., & Cochrane, J. (2015). *The Health of Complex Human Populations*. Washington, DC: National Academy of Medicine.

Sobel, D. (2000). *Galileo's Daughter: A Historical Memoir of Science, Faith and Love*. New York City: Penguin Books.

Wolfe, N. (2011). *The Viral Storm: The Dawn of a New Pandemic Age*. New York: Times Books, Henry Holt and Company.

Step 7

McGaughey, D. R. & Cochrane, J.R. (2017). *The Human Spirit: Groundwork*. Stellenbosch: SUN Press.

Pinker, S. (2011). *The Better Angels of Our Nature: Why Violence Has Declined*. New York: Viking Books.

Pray, L. with Gumm, D. (2012). *Thresholds: Connecting Body and Soul after Brain Injury*. New York: Ruder Finn Press.

Step 8

Higgins, R. (2017). *Thoreau and the Language of Trees*. Oakland, CA: University of California Press.

Acknowledgements

I've listed the names of those in the most immediate learning webs—Stakeholder Health, the Fellows of the Leading Causes of Life Initiative, the colleagues of FaithHealth at Wake Forest Baptist Medical Center and across crazy North Carolina. But seeing the future takes a long memory, so I am constantly strengthened by the heroes of Memphis, the friends at Emory University and The Carter Center, my teachers at Interdenominational Theological Center, the saints of Oakhurst Baptist Church, living and dead, the hearty Seeds people who still stand with the hungry decades on.

What I see through all these eyes is that hope is not delusional and that God is not done. With such a cloud of witnesses, it is almost wrong to name a handful, but even more wrong to not do so: Jim Cochrane, Jerry Winslow, Tom Peterson, Fred Smith, Kevin Barnett, Larry Pray, my daughters Lauren and Kathryn, and of course TC—my best colleague, friend, and wife, without whom I would not see in color and absolutely no numbers at all. I've been transformed through the rich learning ground of Memphis and Winston-Salem, where a shockingly large number of the 25,000 some employees taught me things by word and deed. I hope they see themselves in here.

As I sorted through the bookshelves looking for the sources of some of the citations in the book I found myself gasping at the authors whom I did not cite. How could I write about anything without citing Walter Rauschenbusch or Wendell Berry? How could I write about the human species without a nod to Darwin, or about life without Franz Capra and Stewart Kauffman? How I could I not cite John Nichols, Kelly Carpenter, Lanny Peters, or Mel Williams, all pastors along my learning journey. Just because someone is not cited does not mean they didn't shape the author's mind.

In the preface I said that I identify with those nameless grey cells way back in the brain that struggle to make sense out of the many messages others closer to reality have seen. I am a product of those who have allowed me to see through their eyes, including those who have worked directly with me, especially those at The Carter Center, Emory University, and the FaithHealth divisions of Methodist LeBonheur Healthcare and Wake Forest Baptist Medical Center. Literally thousands of individuals from boardroom to sub-basement have shaped my mind in profound ways. I can think of no thoughts I could claim as only my own.

Two groups deserve to be listed by name. First are the contributing authors of Stakeholder Health whose intellectual generosity in person and at the keyboard knows no bounds. This learning was possible partly because of the financial support of the Investing Partner hospital systems, but no money could buy what the authors gave to my learning process as it did to many others.

Stakeholder Health Authors and Stakeholder Health Advisory Council (SHAC) members

Dustin Aho	Sherrianne Kramer	Margo DeMont
Marice Ashe	Lance Laurence	Nada Dickinson
Bobby Baker	Dory Lawrence	Doug Easterling
Dora Barilla	Sandy Lazarus	Niels French
Kevin Barnett	Marilyn Lynk	Bryan Hatcher
Eileen Barsi	Monica Lowell	Jason Hodges
Caroline Battles	Cheryl McCarver	Heather Wood Ion
Kathie Bender Schwich	Laura McDuffee	Maureen Kersmarki
P. J. Brafford	Jeremy Moseley	Ray King
Pablo Bravo	Kirsten Peachey	Denise Koo
Jane Berz	Cynthia Carter-	Loel Solomon
Ameldia Brown	Perrilliat	Gurmeet Sran
Kenneth Carder	Barb Petee	Tyler Stewart
Heidi Christensen	Catherine Potter	Thomas Strauss
Stephanie Cihon	Tom Peterson	Don Stiger
Joan Cleary	Dominica Rehbein	Soma Stout
Jim Cochrane	Ann Roda	Kimberlydawn
Nancy Combs	Steve Scoggin	Wisdom
Teresa Cutts	Allen Smart	Jerry Winslow
Carla Gober-Parks	Fred Smith	Mark Zirkelbach

And second are the Fellows of the Leading Causes of Life Initiative that have found the bedrock under the ideas. I hope that both groups of colleagues recognize their best thoughts in this book and will forgive the parts I did not understand well enough.

Leading Causes of Life Fellows

Kanwaljeet Anand
Kevin Barnett
Elias Bongmba
Heidi Christensen
Jim Cochrane
Teresa Cutts
Nomvula Dlamini
Doug Easterling
Eugenia Eng
Sharon Engebretsen
Joyce Essien
Shirley Eloby
  Fleming
Ellen Idler
Heather Wood Ion
Evance Kalula
Horst Kleinschmidt

Paul Laurenti
Sandy Lazarus
Jørn Lemvik
Leslie London
Jeremy Moseley
Douglas McGaughey
Malusi Mpumiwana
Shingai Ndinga
Masana Ndinga-Kanga
Bret Nicks
Laura Chanchien
  Parajón
Ken I. Pargament
Jill Olivier
Kirsten Peachey
Tom Peterson
Larry Pray

Doug Reeler
Steve Scoggin
Mohamed Seedat
Rachel Sinha
Fred Smith
Craig Stewart
Soma Stout
Beulah Tertiens-
  Reeler
Anna Tharyan
Herman Tolentino
Emily Viverette
Marlese von
  Broembsen
Francis Wilson
Jerry Winslow

I'm very grateful to Becky De Oliveira and the creative team of Ray Tetz, particularly Alberto Valenzuela, at the Pacific Union Conference who transformed my raw manuscript into the book you hold, a work closer to alchemy than you know. Thanks also to Maria Parries, for her copy editing.

How could I have a page of this work that does not end with a word of love to TC: my wife, friend, colleague, and teacher all along the way.

About the Author

R ev. Dr. Gary Gunderson is Secretary of Stakeholder Health, a learning group of more than 40 healthcare systems engaging their communities to advance health. He represents Stakeholder Health on the Roundtable on Population Health Improvement of the National Academies of Science and serves on the leadership team for 100 Million Healthier Lives. As Vice President for FaithHealth at Wake Forest Baptist Medical Center he leads a division which includes spiritual care, Clinical Pastoral Education, 37 counseling centers and a highly innovative "ground game" focused on the most vulnerable communities across the state. All of this is done in partnerships with hundreds, indeed, thousands, of faith groups through FaithHealthNC. Gary is known for more than two decades of creative work in the field of faith and public health initially at The Carter Center and Emory School of Public Health and then in Memphis, Tennessee, where the ideas found ground through more than 600 congregational partners showing hard evidence of significant improved outcomes including mortality, cost and dramatically lower hospitalization. The work has been cited by JAMA, AHRQ, AHA, IHI, WHO, IOM the White House, HHS and numerous industry venues.

Gunderson is Professor of Public Health Science in the Wake Forest University School of Medicine and Professor of the Health of the Public in the School of Divinity. He is visiting faculty at the University of Cape Town Division of Family Medicine and Public Health where he was one of the founders of the International Religious Health Assets Program.

Gary has authored five books including *Religion and the Health of the Public* with Dr. James Cochrane by Palgrave/McMillian. This was adapted in a version by The Barefoot Collective as *Mobilizing Religious Health Assets for Transformation*, illustrated by Kagan Cochrane. *Deeply Woven Roots*, by Fortress Press has been widely used in seminaries since its publication in 1997. *Boundary Leaders*, also by Fortress, explores the life and work of those working in community and public health. *Leading Causes of Life* by Abingdon Press is anchor of a global network of Fellows exploring the life of institutions and their leaders.

Gary is an ordained American Baptist minister with degrees from Candler School of Theology at Emory University and Doctor of Ministry at the Interdenominational Theological Center in Atlanta as well as an honorary doctorate from the Chicago Theological Seminary. He is married to Dr. Teresa Cutts, also faculty at Wake Forest School of Medicine with four daughters between them: Lauren, Kathryn, Tess and Maya and two grandsons, Charlie and Asa.

92016195R00139

Made in the USA
Middletown, DE
04 October 2018